DATE DUE

OC 29 '93			
AP 18 '94			
AG 18 '94			
MR 6 '95			
NO 9 '95			
MR 29 '96			
OC 14 '97			
NO 30 '98			
NV 18			
NO 2			
FE 10 '00			
JY 18 '01			
NO 15 03			

DEMCO 38-296

KNEE HEALTH

This book aims to explain simply how the knee works, how to protect it from harm, how it can go wrong, what to do and who to see about the problem knee. It is intended to help the child, the pensioner, the sportsman or woman, the worker, the housewife, the leisured person, the active or sedentary person. The book aims to allay any fears, and help people to adopt a logical and positive approach to overcoming, and preventing, knee problems.

While many, if not most, people experience back ache or back pain at some stage in their lives, large numbers also suffer with knee problems. The knees are vital joints for propulsion, balance and shock absorption for any person of any age or sex who walks, runs, crouches, kneels or sits in the course of his or her lifestyle activities.

In sportsmen and women, the knees are generally considered to be the most commonly injured of all the body's joints. Most sports place the harshest stresses on the knee-joints, giving rise to accidents or problems involving mechanical imbalance. Many activities at work, leisure, or in the home pose the same risks to the knees as sports, so non-sporting, active people can suffer similar injuries to sportsmen. Relatively inactive people are not immune to knee problems, some of which can be due to lack of exercise, while others can be accidents very similar to those suffered by sportsmen and women. In older age, the knee-joints can suffer wear-and-tear; in children, growth stresses can magnify minor accidents into more serious knee problems. Diseases, inflammatory conditions and infections can affect the knee-joints in any age group.

Vivian Grisogono has treated knee problems in years of practice as a chartered physiotherapist. In dealing with them, she has worked closely with general practitioner doctors, orthopaedic specialists, rheumatologists, podiatrists and dieticians.

Vivian Grisogono, chartered physiotherapist, is currently in private practice in West London. She has founded the registered Charity, 'Fitness and Rehabilitation Centres Ltd', in order to set up fully equipped, large-scale physiotherapy facilities for the widest range of people who might need them. Although she is now committed to general practice, she has specialized in sports injuries. She set up the first full-time injuries unit at a national sports centre, at Crystal Palace in London, and has attended the World Student Games, Commonwealth Games, Winter Olympics and Summer Olympics as team physiotherapist. She has played tennis and squash to County representative level, and was nationally ranked in squash. She is honorary physiotherapist to the Women's Squash Rackets Association. She lectures regularly to medics, paramedics, coaches and sports participants on safe fitness training and sports injuries. She also contributes magazine articles and broadcasts on those topics. She holds an honorary lectureship to the London Hospital Sports Medicine Diploma Course for doctors. Her book, *Sports Injuries, A Self-Help Guide* (paperback, John Murray) published in 1984, has become a standard work for specialists and sportsmen or women.

Knee Health

Problems, Prevention and Cure

Vivian Grisogono

John Murray

For Andrew, my favourite 'knee patient'

First published 1988
by John Murray (Publishers) Ltd
50 Albemarle Street, London W1X 4BD

Reprinted 1990

Typeset by Fakenham Photosetting Ltd, Fakenham, Norfolk
Printed and bound in Great Britain
by The Bath Press, Avon

British Library Cataloguing in Publication Data

Grisogono, Vivian
    Knee health: problems, prevention
    and cure.
    1. Knee – Wounds and injuries
    I. Title
    617'.582   RD561

    ISBN 0–7195–4386–X

Acknowledgements

Apart from the debt to all my 'knee patients', who have taught me a great deal, special thanks for their help with this book are owed to: Miss Fiona Barr, physiotherapist to the Royal National Orthopaedic Hospital, Stanmore; Mr. Michael Bartlett, artist; Mr. Basil Helal, consultant orthopaedic surgeon; Mr. Roger Hudson, ever-patient editor; Dr. Michael Irani, consultant rheumatologist; Mr. John King, consultant orthopaedic surgeon; Mr. David Kyle, engineer; Mr. Ross Norman, squash player; Mr. Mark Shearman, photographer; and Dr. Neville Sutton, general practitioner.

Contents

1 Who Gets Knee Problems?

While many, if not most, people experience back ache or back pain at some stage in their lives, large numbers also suffer with knee problems. The knees are vital joints for propulsion, balance and shock absorption for any person of any age or sex who walks, runs, crouches, kneels or sits in the course of his or her lifestyle activities. Unfortunately, their versatility makes the knee joints vulnerable to a wide variety of problems. In my practice as a chartered physiotherapist, I have personally treated over 1,200 knee problems in the last eight years. Because of their varied nature, in dealing with them I have worked closely with many different practitioners, including family doctors, orthopaedic surgeons, rheumatologists, podiatrists and dieticians.

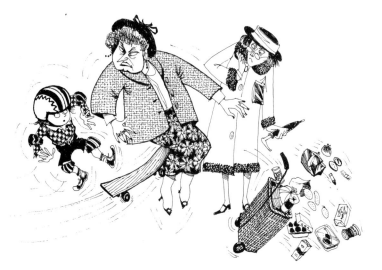

Knees are under constant threat

2. Who Gets Knee Problems?

In sportsmen and women, the knees are generally considered to be the most commonly injured of all the body's joints. Most sports place the harshest stresses on the knee joints, and therefore can lead to accidents, or problems involving mechanical imbalance. Many activities at work, leisure, or in the home pose the same risks to the knees as sports, so active people, although non-sporting, can suffer similar injuries to sports players. Relatively inactive people are not immune to knee problems, as some problems actually arise through lack of exercise. In older age, the knee joints can suffer from wear-and-tear; in children, growth stresses can contribute to knee problems, and can sometimes magnify minor accidents into more serious conditions. Medical problems, including diseases, inflammatory conditions and infections can affect the knee joints in any age group.

The following selected case histories illustrate the variety of problems patients may have, and some lines of treatment a rehabilitation practitioner such as a physiotherapist might apply:

An active twelve-year-old girl, who particularly enjoyed dancing and running, felt her right knee 'click out' when she was practising a new jump in her dance class. This left her with the feeling that two bones were 'rubbing together' over the front of her knee with a grating sensation. The knee was painful if she sat down for long periods (the 'Cinema sign', p. 83), and when she went up and down stairs. Occasionally the knee would 'click out', making walking very painful, but she could ease this by rubbing the knee-cap. She remembered having a similar pain several months previously, following a cross-country run. Although the pain had not been nearly so severe, the knee had felt weak ever since, with a tendency to give way.

Ten days after the injury happened in the dance class, the girl's family doctor referred her for physiotherapy. The lower tip of her knee-cap was tender to touch, as were the fat pads to either side of it, and the tibial tubercle at the top of the shin-bone. The undersurface of the inner side of the knee-cap was sore when pressed. The knee ached if it was bent fully, passively, while she lay on her stomach. Her vastus medialis muscle was extremely weak.

Treatment was aimed at correcting the vastus medialis weakness and the tightness in the quadriceps muscle group, while

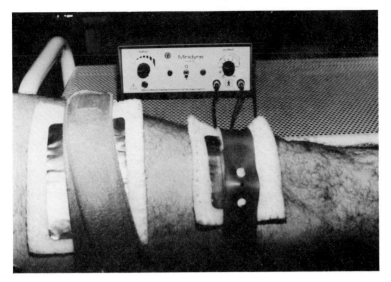

Faradic (electrical) stimulation applied to the vastus medialis muscle

protecting the knee from painful postures and activities. In the first week, she was treated three times with electrical (faradic) stimulation to the vastus medialis muscle, to re-educate the knee's ability to straighten efficiently. There was an immediate improvement in the symptoms. She was not allowed to do any sports, apart from crawl swimming. She had to do knee-straightening exercises and passive quadriceps stretching three times a day, besides trying to straighten her knee frequently whenever she had to sit still for long periods, for instance during school lessons.

In the second week, she was treated three times. Interferential therapy, another kind of electrical treatment, was used for further pain relief. The faradic stimulation was applied not only for static knee-straightening exercises, but also with the knee supported over a pillow, so that it would be straightened from a slightly bent position. By the third week, she was able to do this exercise, with the help of the faradic stimulation, with a light weight over her foot. The vastus medialis weakness was totally corrected. She could bend her knee passively to its full range without discomfort, and riding a bicycle was possible again.

4. Who Gets Knee Problems?

The treatment sessions were not aimed directly at the obvious 'growing problems', such as the chondromalacia patellae or the Osgood-Schlatter's 'disease'. It was considered that most of the girl's pain was due to the poor function of the knee's controlling muscles, which was causing repeated subluxation of the knee-cap. After nine treatment sessions, in the space of three weeks, the girl had no more pain on sitting still or climbing stairs, and she was able to make a gradual return to physical activities. Two years later, she was still painfree.

A 24-year-old professional squash player did his first parachute jump successfully, except that he landed on concrete and 'bounced', bending his left knee inwards. The knee swelled badly, with bruising visible on the inner side of the joint. He attended a hospital casualty department, where it was established that no bone damage was visible on X-ray, and the leg was immobilised in a plaster cast for a week, after which physiotherapy treatment was recommended.

Two weeks after the accident, the knee was still swollen, painful, and very weak, so the patient attended for physiotherapy treatment. He was given one session of faradic stimulation for the grossly weakened vastus medialis muscle, diadynamic therapy for the swelling and pain, and isometric exercises for the thigh. More importantly, he was referred urgently to an orthopaedic consultant at a hospital sports clinic. Three days later he was admitted to hospital, and the consultant operated to repair the torn posterior cruciate ligament in the knee.

Following the operation, the patient spent six weeks in hospital with his leg held bent and the shin-bone held forward in traction by a metal pin. Only a limited amount of movement was allowed in the knee during this period, but daily exercises within those limits were performed to maintain some muscle tone and stimulate the blood flow through the leg. When the patient was finally allowed to get up, his knee was supported in a specially fitted moving splint called the Mackintosh brace, which held the knee so that it could not straighten out fully, nor bend to more than a right angle.

Out of hospital, the rehabilitation programme started eight weeks after the operation. The patient attended for treatment approximately once a week for three months. In the first week, treatment concentrated on manipulating the knee-cap, which was inevitably very stiff, and gently manipulating the knee to help straighten it. A daily exercise programme was set out which included isometric exercises for all the thigh muscle groups, especially the hamstrings; working on an exercise bicycle to strengthen and mobilise the knee, as well as for general fitness; an overall fitness circuit using weights equipment including exercises for the arms and trunk, as well as knee exercises; and swimming, using varied strokes, both for fitness and to improve the injured knee. The patient spent about 2½ hours a day on exercises and training.

In the second week, the treatment session consisted of faradic stimulation to the vastus medialis muscle, and passive stretching manipulations to bend the knee. Balancing on the injured leg and bending the knee slightly was a body-weight-bearing exercise added to the programme. In the third week, faradic stimulation was applied while vastus medialis was worked against weights resistance, straightening the knee through a small range. Balancing on the wobble board was added to the exercise programme, together with intensive feedback exercises for the hamstrings. A minimum of three hours was spent on the daily programme from this point on.

In the sixth week of the programme, the patient started to run for ten minutes, roughly every second day, and he also started solo court practices, simply hitting the squash ball up and down the walls in straight-line patterns. He gradually progressed to running and turning, and then running backwards. After eight weeks, the running was increased to 20 minutes. Lunging exercises were introduced for balance and strength, and court practices with a partner were begun. Shortly afterwards, the player progressed to playing full squash games, and doing court sprints (running, bending and turning in all directions).

Three months after the start of the rehabilitation programme, and five months after the operation, the patient won a squash tournament. Over the next two years, he rose in the world professional ranking lists to number two – higher than before his injury. Three years after the accident, he became world squash champion.

A 43-year-old man in training for the London Marathon woke one morning with pain on the outer side of his left knee. The previous day he had run eight miles in new trainers, which were heavily reinforced in the heel counter and the soles. The marathon was just over three months away. His doctor recommended rest from running for one week, and gave him a cream to rub into the painful area. He then tried to cover three miles alternately jogging and walking, and managed this for three days, but on the fourth day he tried a longer run, and the pain recurred after about two miles. He persevered for another two days, but the pain became too severe, and his knee also stiffened up when he sat down at rest. He therefore took two weeks off running, and his doctor referred him for physiotherapy.

The runner had started long-distance training two years previously. He had completed one marathon and several half-marathons. Following a four-month lay-off due to business commitments, he had built up gradually to running six days a week over a period of five months, averaging roughly forty miles per week, on the basis of five runs over a relatively short distance and one long run per week. Apart from the knee injury, the only problem he had noticed was some back pain after his longer running sessions.

When he attended for physiotherapy assessment and treatment, the tests for the iliotibial tract friction syndrome were positive (see page 121). There was acute tenderness when the outer side of the knee was pressed with the joint held slightly bent. The vastus medialis muscle was weakened. Moreover, the patient had flattened foot arches, and second toes longer than the big toes (Morton's foot), with weight-bearing callouses consequently under the heads of the second toes instead of on the balls of the feet.

Despite the obvious mechanical imperfections in the runner's feet, orthotics were not recommended, because there would have been too little time to have them fitted and get the runner used to them before his event. Moreover, as the problem was obviously triggered by a change to unsuitable running shoes, it was felt that once the inflammation and pain at the side of the knee were cured, the runner should be able to run comfortably, if he reverted to the style of shoe he had been using previously. Therefore all his running shoes were professionally resoled, including the new ones which had caused the problem, which became usable when they were given a softer sole.

Treatment consisted of faradic stimulation to the vastus medialis muscle and separately down the iliotibial tract, to regain good co-ordination on the inner and outer sides of the knee; deep massage over the painful spot on the iliotibial tract; and interferential therapy over the painful area to stimulate it and reduce the soreness. Treatment was applied once a week for five weeks. The patient had to do a daily routine of isometric knee strengthening exercises, with special emphasis on lifting the leg straight upwards with weights. He had to stretch the outer thigh at frequent intervals each day. For more general fitness, and to help his back condition, he did gym work with weights and free exercises, and went swimming.

In the first week of rehabilitation, he went for one run, and managed to complete three miles, although he had some knee pain after one mile. In the second week, he ran four times, and covered over four miles each time, although he was worried that the pain might recur. In the third week, feeling much better and more confident, he ran four times, and covered slightly more distance. In the fourth week he did an eleven-mile run without problems, and in the fifth week he managed fifteen miles in one session. He was instructed to continue his build-up doing three or four running sessions a week, while maintaining his knee exercises and some training in the swimming pool and the gym. Less than six weeks after completing his treatment, he successfully ran in the London Marathon, finishing in a time of five hours – slowed down, not by his knee, but by cramp!

A 46-year-old woman, whose job was child welfare, was sitting down at work when she noticed that her left knee was gradually swelling up until it felt very hot and tight. She had not injured the knee, nor done any unusual activities or movements which might explain the swelling. Her family doctor removed the fluid, but it built up again by the next day. The doctor therefore referred her to a consultant rheumatologist, who tested the patient's blood and urine, and found no evidence of any inflammatory condition. The problem was diagnosed as degenerative arthritis, as the cause was unknown, and the patient was referred for physiotherapy treatment.

When the patient was assessed, six weeks after the knee had swelled up, her knee was still swollen, especially over the front of the joint. She could not squat down because of the tightness in the joint; driving made the knee hurt, and the joint seemed to 'click' when she went up and down stairs. The vastus medialis muscle was weak. When questioned about the background to the injury, the patient remembered that she had fallen down some three years before, injuring the left knee, which swelled up slightly on that occasion. Just two weeks before the knee swelled up badly this time it had swollen slightly, after the patient had spent nearly two hours kneeling down almost continuously while working with young children. The only unusual factor which might have a bearing on the present problem was an especially long walk that she had taken with her dog in the morning before the knee suddenly swelled up. She could not recall any changes in her diet, and her alcohol intake did not vary from one or two glasses of wine each evening, plus an occasional glass of sherry.

Treatment consisted of faradic stimulation for the vastus medialis muscle, massage to the swollen area over the front of the knee, passive stretching techniques for the tight quadriceps muscles, and interferential therapy to help the soreness and swelling. A small patellar strap (see page 86) was used to reduce the knee-cap clicking the patient was noticing on stairs. The patient was instructed to do a daily routine of isometric strengthening exercises for all the thigh muscle groups, passive stretching exercises for the quadriceps muscles, and she was warned against sitting still for too long, twisting her knees while sitting, standing badly, or crouching or kneeling longer than absolutely necessary. After two treatments in the first week, only a little progress seemed to have been made, although the patient said she felt a little better. On the third visit, she remembered that there had been one change in her normal routine: the wine she drank each day was home-made, and she had started drinking a different, cheaper, brand shortly before the knee problem started.

On suspicion that this might have been the triggering factor for an otherwise mysterious problem, the patient was instructed to avoid this type of wine while continuing the knee exercises and the postural care programme already set out. No more physiotherapy treatment was given. Three weeks later, she reported that the swelling had subsided very quickly after this, she was able to squat without pain, stairs were no longer a problem, and the knee felt normal again. The consultant rheumatologist was sceptical that the home-made wine could have been a factor in causing the knee swelling, but the patient has avoided that particular brand ever since, just in case.

An 84-year-old woman was suffering from long-standing pain in her right knee, which had become much worse since she broke her knee-cap four years ago. She had severe osteoarthritis in the knee, and her doctor had discussed the possibility of a knee replacement operation. This was considered impractical because of her age, in view of the trauma and weakening effect involved in the operation, and the time needed to recover from the surgery before regaining full function. As she was, the patient was fully independent and lived alone, managing all her household chores, her shopping, and even a little gardening. She was able to walk, slowly, using a stick. Her problem was the pain in the knee, which became much worse if the knee was being held still, making it difficult for her to get moving when she got out of bed in the morning or stood up after sitting down.

Her family doctor was keeping the problem under control with anti-inflammatory drugs and painkillers, and at intervals he would refer the patient for a course of physiotherapy. The knee was becoming badly deformed, being held bent and bowed. A typical course of physiotherapy consisted of six to twelve weekly sessions of faradic stimulation to improve the vastus medialis muscle; interferential or diadynamic therapy to stimulate the joint and lessen the pain; massage to relieve any swelling and soreness; and passive manipulations to make active movements easier to perform. The patient would be instructed in, and reminded of, the importance of all types of exercise, including isometric exercises for the thigh muscles, gentle mobilising movements to bend and straighten the knee, and some dynamic strengthening exercises. She would also be reminded of correct posture, especially the need to avoid sitting still with the legs crossed or the knees held bent for too long. She was routinely supplied with shock absorbing insoles for her walking shoes.

Treatment usually brought some relief to the knee pain, although this was necessarily temporary. The aim of the treatment was to help the patient maintain her independence for as long as possible, by maintaining the maximum possible strength and mobility in the knee and its muscles.

Many knee problems are preventable, most are curable, but some are only manageable. Understanding the different types of knee problems and their likely consequences can give insights into how to cope with them. Anyone suffering from one of the great variety of possible knee ailments might, understandably, feel confused on first becoming aware of the symptoms. Most people only think of preventing injuries once they have experienced a problem, but personal experience coupled with understanding can be important in preventing re-injury, and perhaps in helping others to avoid similar problems. Parents, for instance, can turn their own knee injury experiences to good advantage by helping their children avoid preventable problems.

2 How Knees Work

The human knee consists of two interlinked joints: the main one links the shin-bone to the thigh-bone, with a subsidiary joint between the knee-cap and the thigh-bone. The knee joints can bend, straighten and twist to either side. Their structure combines strength and stability with a fair degree of mobility. They work hard in many different situations. When we walk, our knees may absorb a pressure equivalent to three times the body weight at every step. In running or landing from a jump, the jarring, or compression, is very much greater. Labourers like hod carriers, who carry heavy weights all day, take a great deal of load through their knees. Carpet-layers, electricians and gardeners who kneel and squat at work put both direct

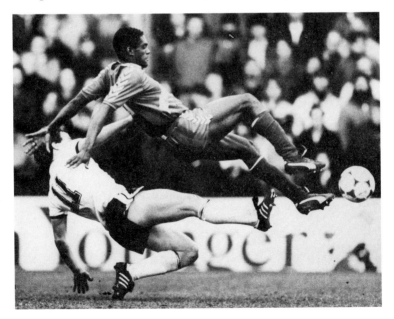

Knees work hard in many different situations

pressure and shearing stress on their knees. Similar pressures occur when house decorators balance on ladders with their knees held at awkward angles. People who drive or sit down in their work incur milder, but significant, shearing stresses in their knees. Many sports stress the knees to their limits, especially games like football which involve running, kicking and direct contact with opponents.

The movements of the human knee are determined by the structural arrangement of bones, capsule, ligaments and muscles which has developed over the millennia of human existence. Within the basic format, knees come in differing shapes and sizes. Our knee joints are outlined at birth, but they change considerably as we grow up and grow old. Knees vary from person to person, and one knee may even be different from the other in one person. These differences are due to many factors: heredity, individual growth patterns, usage, injury and disease can all have an effect on the knee's structural changes and variations. Some of the factors affecting the knee's structural development can be altered or dictated by conscious effort, if we understand the physical effects of our activities and postures, and choose to impose certain patterns of movement on our joints. We have no control over factors like heredity and disease. The configuration of the knee determines its detailed pattern of movement, and can have a bearing on injuries or mechanical problems developing in the joint.

The theoretical 'normal' knee is one in which the shin-bone, in the sideways view, is more or less vertically in line with the thigh-bone in the standing position; the tip of the knee-cap lies

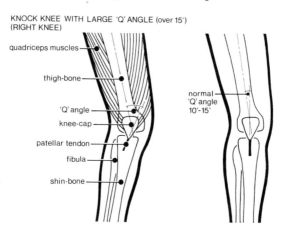

KNOCK KNEE WITH LARGE 'Q' ANGLE (over 15°)
(RIGHT KNEE)

quadriceps muscles

thigh-bone

'Q' angle

knee-cap

patellar tendon

fibula

shin-bone

normal
'Q' angle
10°-15°

over the joint line between the shin and thigh-bones, and the tibial tubercle at the top of the shin lies vertically below the tip of the knee-cap. Seen from the front, the thigh-bone comes down not vertically but diagonally to join the shin-bone at an angle known as the 'Q-angle'. The Q-angle is measured where the line drawn down the centre of the thigh-bone meets the line drawn through the tibial tubercle and patellar tendon. Its normal value is considered to be in the range of 10–15 degrees. If the Q-angle is greater than 15 degrees, it may be due to a very wide pelvis with the hips well apart; a twist on the shin-bone, setting it outwards relative to the thigh-bone; or knock-knees. If the Q-angle value is very small, it may reflect a narrow pelvis with the thigh-bone set more vertically than normal; an inward twist on the shin-bone; or bow legs.

Many of the different shapes that knees can form have descriptive names and are easily recognizable. Knees which bend inwards towards each other are called knock-knees, and the technical term for them is genu valgum. Knees which bend outwards, away from each other, are called bow legs, with the technical name genu varum. Knees which curve backwards, or hyperextend, are technically termed genu recurvatum. If the knees are slightly bent, seen from the side, and cannot straighten out to put the shin-bone in line with the thigh-bone, the knee is said to be held in fixed flexion: if the knees are very bent, the description is fixed flexion deformity. When the knee-caps are positioned noticeably high in relation to the knee joints, the technical term is patella alta.

GENU RECURVATUM WITH PATELLA ALTA (RIGHT LEG OUTER SIDE)

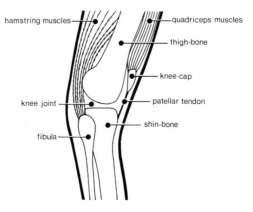

14. How Knees Work

The knees are part of a co-ordinated mechanism involving all the joints and muscles of the legs. If the feet are flat (pes planus), or tend to roll inwards and over-pronate, pressure is created on the inner sides of the knees and this can contribute to knock-knees. Feet with high arches (pes cavus) which roll outwards, over-supinating, stress the outer sides of the knees, and can have a bearing on bow legs. Stiff ankles can cause compensatory over-mobility in the knees. Shoes which limit foot movements or create faulty movements can also affect the knees badly: very high heels, for instance, alter the body's balance and the walking pattern, and can create abnormal stresses over the knees. If a person has one leg longer than the other, the knee alignment may be different on each leg. Turned-in hips can be a factor in knock-knees. If the hips are set very wide apart, they can contribute to hyperextended knees. If the hamstring or calf muscles are tight, the knee may be pulled into the fixed flexion position. If the quadriceps group is excessively strong compared to the hamstrings, the hamstrings may be unable to stabilize the shin-bone properly from behind.

The human body has developed in relation to gravity's pressure, and much of its structure is dictated by this. Our legs are much more solid than our arms, because they support our body's weight against gravity all the time that we are upright on our feet, whereas our arms are no longer used much for body support in normal life. When a person is standing still, the human body has its own centre of gravity, which is theoretically roughly in front of the upper part of the sacrum at the back of the pelvis. The line of gravity passes from the top of the head down through the midline of the body to between the feet, just in front of the line of the ankle joints. The body has to work continually to hold itself upright against gravity's downward pressure. Our balance mechanisms dictate automatic muscular adjustments, if there is a slight body sway during standing. Round the knees, the quadriceps work to prevent the joints from folding under gravity's pressure, and the other thigh muscles come into action if needed. We are not normally aware of this muscle activity, and the knees feel quite relaxed while we stand still.

When we consciously activate our knee muscles, we can create different types of muscle work. By tensing up a muscle group without creating movement in a joint, we work the muscles isometrically or statically. When we use our muscles to create knee movements, they work dynamically. The muscles may shorten in order to create the movement against gravity or some other type of resistance: this is called concentric contraction. If the muscles are working in the same direction as gravity, or resisting a pulling force, they lengthen out to exert control, and this is called eccentric muscle work. Like any other joint, the knee has an arc, or range, of movement, and its muscles' efficiency alters according to which part of the movement they are working in. A muscle group is at a disadvantage when it works with its fibres shortened: this is called inner range muscle work. For instance, it is very hard to bend the knee fully with the leg stretched back from the hip, because the hamstrings are fully shortened. The middle part of the range is usually the strongest, but a muscle can be stimulated to a powerful contraction by stretching its fibres out fully before it is activated. Muscle groups automatically co-ordinate with each other during conscious, or voluntary, movements, so that while one muscle group is contracting to create a movement its opposite group relaxes, while other groups may act to stabilise surrounding joints.

Most human movements and physical activities involve a combination of different types of muscle work, together with an element of fitness, even in the most inactive or un-sporting person. Strength is a muscle's ability to generate force; endurance, or stamina, is its ability to generate that force repeatedly; power is the muscle's ability to generate force in a unit of time, i.e. at speed. Any normal activity may be limited by muscle weakness or lack of stamina. Reaching up to a high shelf may involve standing on tiptoe, holding the knee muscles in isometric contraction: lack of muscle strength and endurance may mean that the person can only spend a few seconds at a time in this position, whereas a trained ballet dancer can hold the position on one leg without effort. A short sprint for a bus involves muscle power for speed, a longer run requires endurance: lack of fitness may mean missing the bus.

Walking up and down stairs is a normal activity which reflects how varied human movement can be through fitness factors. Going up stairs, the weak person bends forwards, saving energy by lowering the body's centre of gravity and using the propulsive muscles, mainly the quadriceps group, in their strong middle range. The effort may still cause puffing and panting by the top of the flight, if muscle endurance is very poor. A stronger person is likely to stand straighter, and to straighten the legs at each step. A fit sports player may sprint up the stairs and not be short of breath. Coming down stairs is harder on the muscles than going up, as it involves eccentric loading through the leg muscles, especially the quadriceps group. If the muscles are very weak, the knees tend to buckle and give way.

The knees are constructed for physical activity, and their muscles become weak through lack of use. Inactivity is as bad for the knees as bad movements or overuse. Muscle imbalance and joint defects can be brought on by sitting still for long periods, allowing the knees to stiffen, and habitually standing or sitting in poor postural alignment. For instance, standing with the weight balanced over one knee, holding the other slightly bent, tends to overload the weight-bearing knee and distort the other. Sitting with the legs twisted at awkward angles may stress the knee ligaments. Both types of bad posture undermine the balance of muscles round the knee. Good posture is based on body symmetry.

3 How to Protect the Knees

• **Keep active.** The knees need movement, to keep the joint mechanisms lubricated, and the muscles in good working order. Staying still for long periods is bad for the knees, and should be avoided. In a job which involves sitting all day, it is usually possible to stand up at intervals, and perhaps walk around. Schoolchildren, students and secretaries at their desks can straighten their knees out periodically, either by lifting each heel off the floor in turn, or by stretching each leg out to place the foot on the floor and straighten the knee back. People who have to kneel and crouch in their jobs, like carpet-layers and plumbers, should stand up frequently and stretch their legs.

Even very small movements can help to give the knees cyclical exercise and prevent joint stiffness. People who have to stand still for long periods, such as soldiers and shop assistants, can benefit from moving their knees very slightly, bending and straightening the joints.

Anyone confined to bed for a long time through illness should exercise the knees as fully and as often as possible, preferably turning onto each side and onto the stomach, to exercise all the leg muscles, and prevent skin pressure problems. Circulatory flow is important for everyone, but stimulating blood flow through the legs is especially important to the person on bed-rest, to prevent blood clots from forming.

• **Maintain the knees' full movements.** Most everyday activities do not use the whole of the knees' possible range of movement. In walking, for instance, the knees only bend and straighten slightly, although they bend more going up or down stairs. The axiom 'if you don't use it, you lose it' applies to joint mobility as well as muscle strength. Therefore, to prevent joint stiffness, it is advisable to bend and straighten the knees fully a few times a day. Mobilising exercises, like those on pp. 30–33, help to keep the knees free-moving, while stretching exercises (pp. 33–35) prevent any muscular stiffness round the joints.

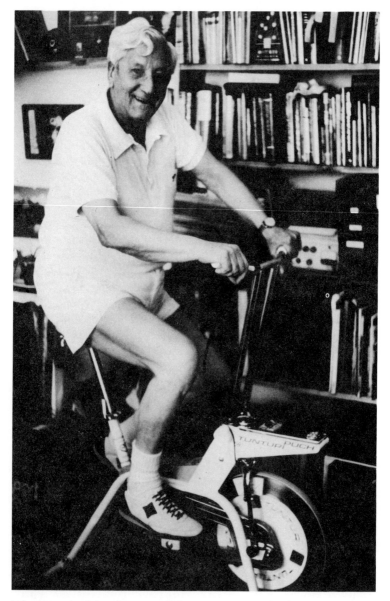

The exercise bicycle, a good 'home exercise' for knees, demonstrated by the Author's father, aged 74

- **Maintain good muscle balance round the knees.** Muscle strength and flexibility can be improved at any age through exercises. Everyday movements can be made into protective exercises, for instance getting up from a chair or sitting down on it using the leg muscles, instead of leaning on the hands. While standing still, the thigh muscles can be tensed for a few seconds at a time, to tighten the knee-caps.

  Anyone who has a physically demanding job, or is involved in active sports, should do protective exercises as essential background training. Isometric exercises, like those on pp. 24–27, stabilise the knees, and should be done on a daily basis. Dynamic exercises (pp. 35–38) provide strength through ranges of movement. All the knee's surrounding muscles should be worked in turn: if one area is particularly weak or tight, extra work should be done to improve it.

  Weight training is especially valuable in providing a progressive system for improving the muscles. Fixed-weight systems like Nautilus, Norsk, David, Schnell, Universal and Powersport are easy to use and provide exercises for all the major muscle groups in the leg, using a good range of joint movement. Muscles can be toned up, improving strength and stamina without any increase in size, or bulked up, according to the number of repetitions and degree of loading used in the exercises. Weight training should be part of the general conditioning programme for any sport, but it can also be enjoyable and beneficial for non-sporting people.

- **Avoid harmful movements.** Lifting heavy loads or carrying weights all day may over-stress the knees, especially if the muscles round the joints are weak. It is important to use the knees when lifting a heavy weight, to protect the back from over-straining. For a correct lift, the knees should bend evenly, while the back is held locked straight; the load is kept as close to the body as possible, and the legs provide the upward propulsion to lift it off the ground. Anyone who has to lift or place loads at awkward angles, for instance in landscape gardening or the building trade, should have helpers to lessen the strain. If possible, the work of lifting or carrying heavy loads should be spaced out to give the knees 'rest periods' where they can be moved or exercised without load. If the knees are not strong enough to cope with work like heavy labouring, it may be necessary to consider changing jobs.

20. How to Protect the Knees

Repetitive jarring or compression can overload the knees. The marathon runner on a high mileage training schedule is an example of a person at risk of this kind of overload. To protect the knees, the marathoner should vary the training schedule, running at different speeds, on different kinds of terrain, and including protective conditioning exercises for the whole body, with special emphasis on the leg muscles, on a daily basis. Shock-absorbing polymer insoles are useful to marathoners and to soldiers who have to run and march in hard boots. This type of insole can also help to reduce jarring stresses from walking in leather-soled shoes on hard pavements.

Using the knees bent, without straightening the joints, can upset the mechanical balance of muscles round the knees. Any knee-bending activity should be balanced by knee-straightening movements or exercises (pp. 24–27). A driver should make sure that the car seat is as far back as possible, to allow the legs to straighten onto the pedals. If the car seat slopes downwards at the back, a cushion raising the level will allow the driver's legs to straighten out. On a bicycle, the rider should have the seat as high as is safe, so that the knees are almost straight on the downward sweep of the pedal. The rider should remember to stand up in the pedals when cycling up a hill.

Any movement or activity which brings on pain or swelling in the knees should be avoided. The cause of such symptoms must be identified, so help should be sought from the doctor or specialist. Sometimes extreme fatigue or viral infections can make the knees and other joints ache, giving the first warning that the person should be resting for recovery. When the symptoms are associated with a particular activity, it may be possible to modify the activity and continue on a limited scale: for instance the long-distance runner may be able to run shorter distances, such as half-marathons or ten-kilometres, when marathon running and training cause knee pain.

- **Avoid sudden changes of routine.** A sudden heavy lift can overload the knees and the back, so a weightlifter or manual worker must build up progressively to lifting or carrying heavier weights, to ensure that the body is strong enough to cope. A long walk can over-stress the knees, in the person who normally leads a sedentary life, whereas the person who normally walks a lot can usually cope easily with a longer walk than usual.

In sports, the principle of conditioning the body to cope with stress applies to every session of a sporting activity. The body should be prepared for every training or playing session with a warm-up, which is especially important if the weather is cold, or for the person who has previously been sitting down for long periods, such as the office worker who plays a game in the evening. In the longer term, the body needs to be conditioned gradually to a sporting activity, therefore anyone new to a sport should start by playing only a little, and only once or twice a week. Technique should be learned properly, preferably from an effective coach. If a player takes on a fitness training schedule, it should be based on gradual progression, and should include rest days for recovery.

• **Use cushioning or padding.** When the knees are subjected to direct pressure, the joints should be protected. People who have to kneel should use kneeling pads or cushions. Players of contact sports like American football, or whose sport involves a high risk of falling on the knees, like skateboarding, should

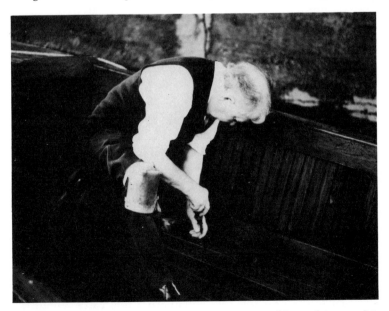

Carpet layer's kneeling pads for an 84-year-old working on his boat

wear padded, properly fitted knee cushioning to absorb shock.

Knee pads worn round the joints have to be broad and thick enough to provide good protection, but they also have to allow for free movement, and the straps have to hold the pads firmly in place without constricting the skin.

• **Wear suitable shoes.** Slippery soles on an icy pavement can cause falls. Very firm, thick rubber-soled shoes or boots are normally needed for heavy labouring jobs, to provide good grip underfoot and protection over the top of the feet. In sports, shoes should be appropriate to the playing surface, so studs are used in field games, spikes on a running track, non-slip rubber soles on synthetic fields and indoor surfaces, and smoother soles for carpet surfaces such as some indoor tennis courts.

Very rigid shoes or badly shaped soles and uppers interfere with normal foot and ankle movements, and can cause secondary stresses through the knees. Foot movements which are faulty in themselves can be corrected by specially fitted inserts, or orthotics, made to measure by a podiatrist. If high heeled shoes are worn for long periods, barefoot walking or flat heels are recommended, to allow the leg muscles to stretch back to normal. High heels should not be worn by very young girls, because they alter the body's normal balance, causing stresses in the legs and lower back which can damage the joints during the delicate growth phases, especially in the early teenage years.

For shoes which are hard or thin in the sole, or if added protection is needed from jarring stresses during walking, running or jumping, polymer shock-absorbing insoles can reduce the compression forces which might otherwise be taken through the knees. Foam rubber or cellular material insoles can provide sufficient protection, if the soles are only slightly hard, or the compression effects not too great.

• **Recover fully from injury.** If a knee is used for normal activities too soon after an injury, it is likely to be re-injured, or a secondary injury may occur in an associated joint or muscle. Following any injury, the process of rehabilitation must be taken through its various stages. Full recovery means a return to normal strength and movement. In a few cases where the knee injury has been specially severe, full recovery may not be possible, so it may be necessary to wear a brace, preferably individually fitted, for potentially stressful activities like skiing. Occasionally, if the injured knee has remained very unstable despite remedial exercises, a supportive brace may be needed for all normal activities, and stressful sports have to be avoided altogether.

• **Maintain good posture.** Standing or sitting awkwardly distorts the knee joints, besides putting abnormal pressures on the hips and lower back. Slouching, turning one foot out or in relative to the other, sitting with one leg crossed over the other, or sitting with the feet tucked sideways at awkward angles are all postures to be avoided. Standing and sitting comfortably straight, keeping an even, symmetrical balance between each side of the body, allows the body's weight to be distributed evenly through all the load-bearing joints, including the knees.

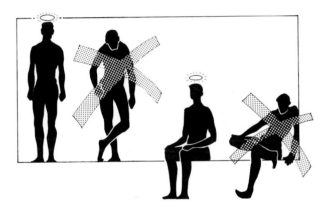

4 Protective and Remedial Exercises

EXERCISES WITH THE KNEE HELD STRAIGHT: THE
STATIC (ISOMETRIC) QUADRICEPS REGIME

1. Knee-cap twitch. Stand with the knees straight but relaxed. Tighten one thigh, to pull the knee-cap upwards, keeping the knee straight. Do the movement slowly at first, then try to flicker the thigh muscles rapidly, to twitch the knee-cap several times. Do ten to twenty twitches on each knee in turn. This exercise can also be done sitting on the floor.

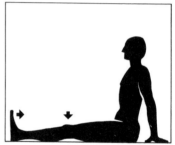

2. Sit on the floor, with your legs straight in front of you. Tighten up the thigh muscles to press the knees downwards into the floor, while pulling your toes back from the ankles so they point upwards; hold for three, then relax completely. This exercise can also be done standing up, locking the knees back as straight as they can go. Repeat ten times, exercising both knees together, or each in turn if one is much weaker than the other.

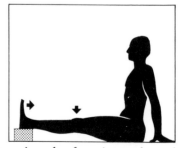

3. Sit on the floor with your legs straight, and your heels resting on a small block, rolled towel or cushion. Press your knees downwards towards the floor, pointing your toes upwards, hold for three, then relax. Repeat ten times, both knees together, or each in turn. This exercise can be varied by turning the foot inwards and straightening the knee, and then turning the foot outwards and repeating the movement.

4. Lie on one side, lock your knees straight, and lift your uppermost leg straight up sideways, keeping your hip well forward, so that your leg is slightly behind you; hold for three, slowly lower. Repeat ten times, then turn over and lift the other leg sideways. Grad-

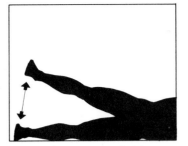

ually add in increasing weight-resistance, by means of either an ankle strap or a weights-boot on the foot.

5. Lie on your stomach (over a pillow if this is more comfortable), lock one knee straight, and lift that leg straight up backwards just a little way, with your toes pointed down away from you; hold for three, slowly lower. Repeat ten times, then repeat on the other leg. Gradually add in weights.

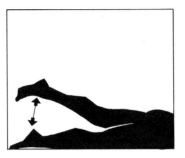

6. Lie on your stomach, lock both knees straight, and lift both legs a little way backwards; separate your legs to take them sideways, hold for three, then slowly lower. Repeat ten times. Gradually add in weights.

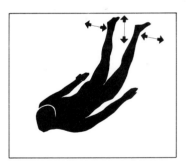

7. Lie on your stomach, tuck your toes under your feet, and straighten your knees hard to lift them backwards, so that you rest on your hips and your toes; hold for three, slowly lower. Repeat ten times, both legs together, or ten on each leg in turn.

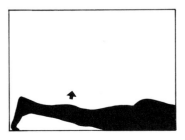

8. Lie on your stomach, with your hands behind your head, legs straight; lift your arms, head, shoulders and one leg a little way backwards, lower, then lift your arms and head with the other leg. Repeat twenty times. Gradually add in leg weights.

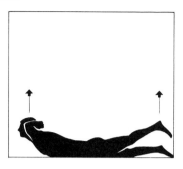

9. Sit on the floor with your legs straight; lock one knee hard, and lift that leg straight upwards; hold for a count of three, slowly lower. Repeat ten times, each leg. Gradually add in weights.

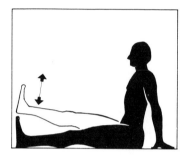

10. Sit on the floor with your legs straight; lock one knee hard and lift that leg to trace the alphabet in the air. Repeat the process with the other leg.

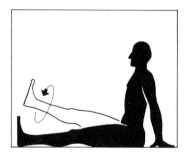

11. Lie on your back with your legs straight; lock one knee, lift the leg straight up in the air a little way, take the leg out sideways, then in across the other leg, back to centre, then slowly lower. Ten times, each leg. Gradually add in weights.

12. Lie on your side with your elbow under your shoulder, forearm at right angles to your body; lift your hips straight up sideways so that you are balanced on your elbow and feet, hold for three, slowly lower. Repeat ten times, then turn onto the other side and repeat.

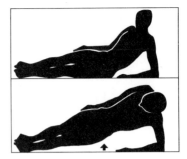

EXERCISES WITH THE KNEE HELD BENT: THE HAMSTRING-EMPHASIS EXERCISE PROGRAMME

1. Lying on your stomach with the knee bent at a right angle, lift the leg a little way backwards, hold for three, slowly lower. Repeat ten times, or build up to fifty quick repetitions. Gradually add weights, over the thigh.

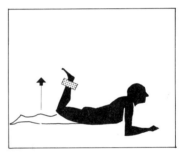

2. Lying on your stomach with your knee bent to a right angle, lift the leg backwards, take it out sideways, back to centre, slowly lower. Build to three sets of ten, then gradually add in weights.

3. Lying on your side with the injured knee uppermost, lift the leg up sideways, holding the hip well forward, so the leg is held slightly behind the trunk; hold for three, slowly lower. Build up to three sets of ten, then add weights resting on the thigh just above the knee.

4. Sit in a chair with the knee bent to a right angle; lift the knee straight up, hold for three, then slowly lower. Build up to three sets of ten, then add weights resting on the thigh just above the knee.

5. Stand on your uninjured leg, with your knees level, injured knee bent. Take your injured leg backwards a little way, hold for three, lower back. Build up to three sets of ten.

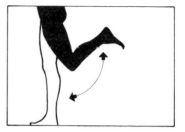

6. Sit in a chair with knees bent; gently tighten the muscles in your injured leg, as though you were trying to press your heel back. Hold for a count of five, then relax completely. Once the cast is removed, this exercise can be done by pressing the heel against the chair leg. Repeat up to ten times.

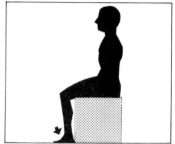

7. Sitting in a chair, gently tighten the muscles in your injured leg, as though you were trying to press your foot outwards. Hold for a count of five, relax completely. When the cast is removed, press the outer border of the foot against the chair leg for resistance. Repeat up to ten times.

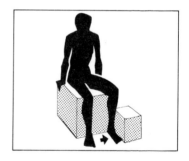

8. Sitting in a chair, gently tighten your injured leg muscles as though you were pulling your heel backwards and turning your foot outwards at the same time. Hold for five, relax completely. With the cast off, do this exercise against an immovable resistance at the back of the heel and the side of the foot. Repeat up to ten times.

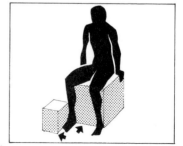

9. Lying on your stomach with a weight over your foot, bend your knee to bring your heel to your seat, then slowly lower back until your knee is at an angle of roughly thirty degrees, i.e. not quite straight. Repeat ten times, gradually increasing the weight. This exercise can be done on a hamstring curl machine, provided that you use your uninjured leg to move the weight from the fully extended position.

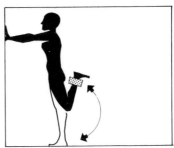

10. Stand on your uninjured leg, with your injured knee slightly bent with a weight strapped to the ankle. Bend your injured knee up behind you, keeping your hip well forward, slowly lower back to the original position. Ten times, then gradually increase the weight.

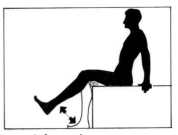

11. Sit on a high chair or stout table, with a rolled towel supporting your injured knee, and a weight over the ankle. Straighten the knee to about thirty degrees from full extension, hold for three, then slowly lower. Build up to three sets of ten, then gradually increase the weight-resistance.

MOBILISING EXERCISES TO BEND AND STRAIGHTEN
THE STIFF KNEE

1. Sit on a table or high chair, with your stiff leg straight in front of you supported on your other leg. Very gently let your uninjured leg bend, until you reach the limit of movement in your stiff knee. Rock your knees gently backwards and forwards at this point, without 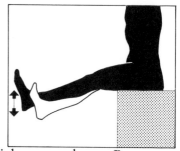 forcing the movement, then straighten your knees. Repeat ten times, increasing to three sets of ten.

2. Lying on your back, bend your injured knee onto your chest. With your hands holding your shin just below the knee, gently pull your knee towards your chest in a bouncing movement. Repeat ten times, building up to three sets of ten.

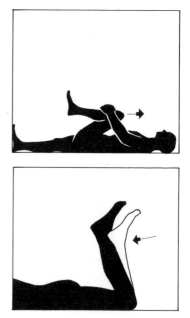

3. Lying on your stomach, with the heel of your uninjured leg resting on the front of the shin on your injured leg, push back with your good leg to bend your knees, pressing your heels towards your seat in a rhythmical bouncing movement. Repeat ten times, increasing to thirty.

4. Sitting on the floor with your foot resting on a polished linoleum surface sprinkled with talcum powder, gently slide your heel backwards and forwards over the smooth surface, letting your knee gradually bend further. This exercise can also be done sitting on a low stool with a roller skate on the foot to allow a free gliding movement. Repeat ten times, building up to five sets of ten.

5. Lying on your stomach, bend your injured knee and hold your ankle in your hand. Pull your foot gently towards your seat, rocking the foot backwards and forwards to bend the knee comfortably to its limit. Repeat ten times, building up to three sets of ten.

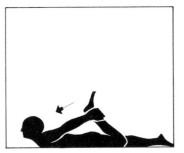

6. Standing on your uninjured leg, rest your injured knee on a chair, with a pillow under it for comfort. Gently rock your seat back to your heel, to bend the knee. Repeat ten times.

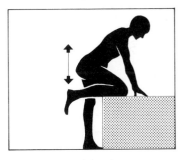

7. Holding onto a bar or support at shoulder height with both hands, gently bend your knees in a bouncing movement until you are squatting down as far as your knee will bend. Straighten your legs, then repeat the squatting movement five times. Do this exercise in

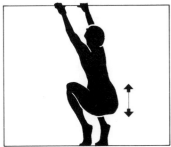

front of a mirror, if possible, to make sure the movement is symmetrical.

8. Sit on a chair, with your injured knee bent as far as it will go, and your foot flat on the floor. Keeping the heel on the ground, turn your toes inwards six times, then outwards, to twist the knee slightly. Then try to bend your knee a little further back. Repeat the process three times.

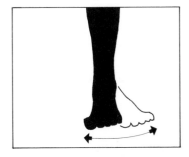

9. On an exercise bicycle, set the saddle to a level just below the point at which you can turn the pedal fully with your injured knee. With no resistance, keep pushing the pedal rhythmically backwards and forwards to the limit of the knee's bending movement, until you can make a full turn. Then lower the saddle slightly and repeat the process.

10. Breast-stroke swimming can help the knee's bending movements. Exercises can be done in the pool too, for instance holding the rails when facing the side of the pool, and gently bending your knees to swing your legs upwards towards your chest, then straightening your legs out behind you.

11. Lie on your stomach on the end of a bed, couch or table, with your knees and lower legs unsupported over the end. Let your legs relax to straighten your knee as far as it can go. Hold the position for a count of ten, then bend your knee. Repeat five times.

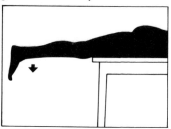

12. Sit on the floor, with a strong belt or rolled towel looped under the ball of the foot on the stiff leg. Keeping the knee as straight as possible, pull the ends of the belt or towel towards you to pull the foot upwards and straighten the knee fully. Hold for a count of five, then relax. Repeat five times.

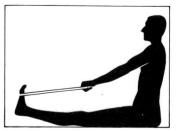

13. Lie on your stomach with your knees and lower legs over the end of the bed, table or couch, and attach a weight to your ankle or a weight boot to your foot. Let your knee lower slowly to its straightest position, relax for a count of five, then bend the knee quickly before lowering it back slowly and holding the straightened position again. Repeat ten times, and build up to three sets of ten.

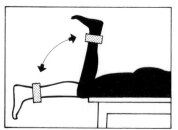

14. Sit on the floor with legs straight and a small support, such as a book, under the heel of the stiff leg. Press the knee downwards to straighten it in a rhythmical bouncing movement, ten times, building up to fifty. Then repeat the exercise with a weight lying over the lower thigh just above the knee.

15. Lie on your stomach on the floor with a support, for instance a folded towel, under your lower thigh just above your knee, and tuck your toes under so that your legs are balanced on the balls of the feet. Press your stiff knee straight to try to lift it away from the support, in a rhythmical bouncing movement. Repeat ten times quickly, building to twenty.

MUSCLE STRETCHING EXERCISES

1. Calf stretch. With one leg behind the other, feet in line, back heel flat on floor, gently bend forward knee, so that you feel a pulling sensation on calf of hind leg. Hold position still for a count of ten, slowly release. Repeat on the other leg, five times each leg.

2. Double calf stretch. Lean forwards against a wall. Move your legs backwards, keeping your heels flat on the floor, until you feel the pull on both calves. Hold for ten, slowly release. Repeat five times.

3. Front thigh stretch. Standing on one leg, bend the other knee up, to hold your ankle behind you with your hand. Pull your heel towards your seat, keeping your hip well forward, until you feel the stretch on the front of your thigh. Hold for ten, then repeat on the other leg, five times on each leg.

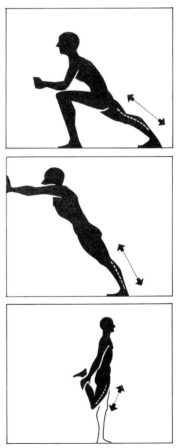

4. Single or double front thigh stretch. Lying on your stomach, bend one or both knees, holding your ankle(s) in your hand(s). Press your heel(s) gently towards your seat, hold for ten, then gently release. Repeat five times.

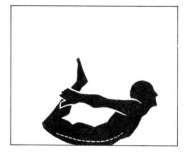

5. Hamstring stretch. Sitting on the floor with your legs straight out in front of you, reach forward to hold your ankles or feet with your hands, bending at the hips and keeping your back as straight as possible, and your head up. Hold for ten, gently release. Repeat five times.

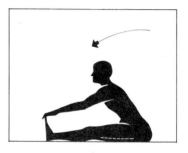

6. Single hamstring stretch. Stand on one leg, resting the other leg comfortably on a support straight in front of you. Reach forward from the hips to hold your ankle or foot with your hand, keeping your back straight, head up. Hold for ten, then repeat on the other leg, five times each leg.

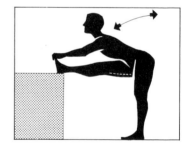

7. Inner thigh stretch. Standing with your legs apart, shift your weight over one hip, and lean sideways over the other leg, until you feel the stretch on the inner thigh you are leaning over. Hold for a count of ten, gently release. Repeat five times on each leg.

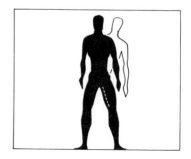

8. Inner thigh stretch. Sitting with your legs stretched as far apart as possible, knees straight, gently bend forward from the hips, keeping your back straight, to feel the stretch on the inside of your thighs. Hold for ten, repeat five times.

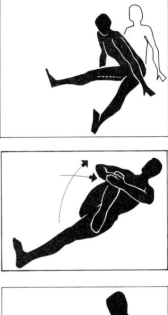

9. Outer thigh stretch. Lying on your back or standing up, bend your knee up towards your chest, and pull the knee towards the opposite shoulder with your hands. Hold for ten, gently release. Repeat five times on each leg.

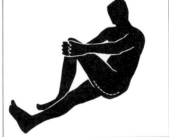

10. Outer thigh stretch. Sitting on the floor with one leg straight, bend the other knee to put your foot on the floor beside the straight knee. Pull the bent knee across the other leg with your hands, to feel the stretch on the outer thigh. Hold for ten. Do five on each leg.

DYNAMIC STRENGTHENING EXERCISES

1. Sit with your legs in front of you, with a cushion or rolled towel under your knee, and a light weight over your ankle. Straighten your knee hard, hold for two, slowly lower. Build up to three sets of ten on each leg, with gradually increasing weights.

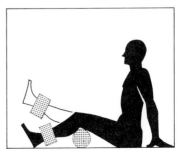

2. Sit with your legs straight in front of you, bend one knee, keeping your heel on the floor, then straighten up the knee to lift your foot in the air. Slowly lower the leg, keeping your knee straight. Build up to three sets of ten on each leg, then add in gradually heavier weights.

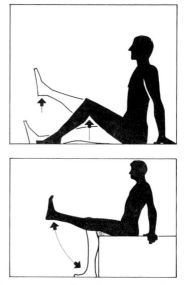

3. Sit on a chair or high table, with a rolled towel or cushion under your knees, and a light weight over your foot or ankle. Straighten your knee fully, hold for two, slowly lower. Build up to three sets of ten on each leg, then gradually in-

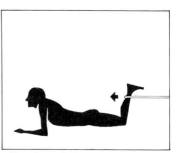

crease the weights. This exercise can also be done on a leg extension machine in a fixed-weights system.

4. Lie on your stomach, with your legs straight, and a weight over your foot or ankle. Bend your knee fully, slowly lower back, keeping your hips flat on the floor. Build up to three sets of ten on each leg, then grad- ually increase the weights. This exercise can also be done

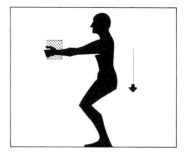

on a hamstring curl machine in a fixed-weights system.

5. Stand, keeping your back as straight as possible. Slowly bend your knees to just beyond a right angle, then rapidly straighten your knees, locking them out. Build up to three sets of ten, adding gradually in- creasing weights, held in your hands or over your shoulders.

6. Repeat exercise 5, on one leg at a time.

7. Sit on a low chair or stool, with your feet parallel and slightly apart, your arms folded across your chest. Stand up, keeping your back straight, then bend your knees slowly to touch the chair lightly with your seat, repeating the movement in quick succession. Build up to three sets of ten, then add in weights, held in the hands.

8. Repeat exercise 7, on one leg at a time.

9. Stand in front of a bench (or double stairs), about 15–20 inches high. Step up onto the bench, straightening your knees fully, then down, in quick succession. Lead with one leg for one set of movements, then change for the second set. Build up to three sets of ten on each leading leg.

10. Using the leg press machine in a fixed weights system, bend and straighten your knees fully, building up to three sets of ten, and then gradually increasing the weights.

11. Use a rowing machine, starting with five minutes at a light resistance, and gradually building up to twenty minutes against an increasing resistance.

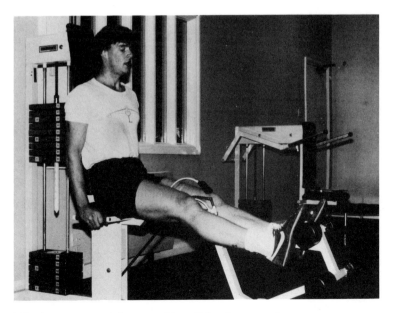

The leg press weights machine (Norsk system)

12. On an exercise bicycle, adjust the saddle height so that your leg is almost straight on the downward sweep of the pedal. Set the resistance to a moderate tension, and pedal at a constant speed for up to five minutes. Gradually increase the resistance, and build up to twenty minutes.

FUNCTIONAL (FINAL REHABILITATION) EXERCISES
FOR EVERYDAY LIFE

1. Sitting on an upright chair, stand up, then slowly sit down again, using your legs only and not your arms. Repeat three to five times, two or three times a day. Make the exercise harder by using a lower chair or sofa.

2. Stand on one leg and hold your balance, timing yourself to see how long you can stand absolutely still. Repeat on the other leg. Try to hold your balance a little longer each time. When the exercise is easy, try balancing with your eyes closed. Repeat once or twice a day.

3. Lying on your back with your knees bent, feet flat on the floor, lift your hips up to balance on your shoulders and feet, then slowly lower. Repeat ten times, once or twice a day.

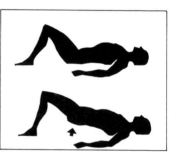

4. Standing on one leg with your back to a strong table, bend your knee a little way to touch your seat gently to the table, then straighten up quickly. Do five to ten movements in quick succession, then repeat on the other leg, once or twice a day.

5. In the swimming pool, swim, using any stroke, and trying to increase your speed or distance at each session. In the shallow end, try walking in the water, first forwards, then sideways and backwards. If you enjoy swimming, try to go at least once a week, regularly.

6. Standing facing a wall, just in front of it, stretch up on your toes and stretch your arms upwards to see how high you can reach on the wall. Hold for a count of two, then relax. Repeat three times, once or twice a day.

7. Standing, holding a support, bring one leg straight up in front of you as high as you can, then swing the leg backwards and bend the knee to try to touch your heel towards your seat, keeping your back straight. Repeat five times on each leg, once or twice a day.

8. Stand facing a step or the lowest stair, holding the rail if necessary. Step up onto the stair, straightening your knee, then step down with the same leg. Repeat five times, leading with one leg, then change to lead with the other, once or twice a day. Then repeat the exercise backwards, stepping onto the stair backwards and coming down forwards.

9. Walk forwards and backwards, for ten to twenty paces. Then walk sideways in each direction, taking your leg first in front of the other leg, then behind it. Then walk in each direction, making sudden turns to one side or the other. Repeat two or three times a day.

10. Barefoot, walk on your toes, for ten to twenty steps; then walk on the outer edges of your feet; then the inner edges; finally on your heels. Build up to three sets of twenty steps, once or twice a day.

FUNCTIONAL (FINAL REHABILITATION) EXERCISES FOR SPORTS

1. Alternate leg thrusts. Crouching on the floor, resting on your hands, with your legs straight behind you, bend one knee up to your chest, then kick that leg out behind you, while you bend the other knee up to your chest, in quick succession. Start with ten movements on each leg, and build up to fifty.

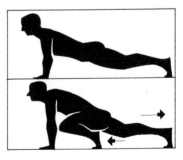

2. Squat thrusts. As exercise 1, but bending and kicking both legs together. Start with ten, build up to three sets of ten.

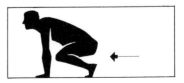

3. Burpees. Bend your knees as for the squat thrust, but jump upwards after bending your knees to your chest, then spring down to kick your legs back behind you. Build up to three sets of ten.

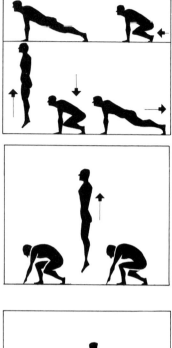

4. Squat jumps. Stand with one foot slightly in front of the other. Jump down, to touch your hands to the floor, then spring up, changing your foot position in the air, so that you land with the hind foot forward. Repeat the movement in quick succession, building up to three sets of ten.

5. Bench jumps. Stand over a bench, with your feet on either side of it. Jump up to touch your heels together in the air over the bench, landing with feet on either side of the bench. Repeat the jumps in quick succession, building up to three sets of ten.

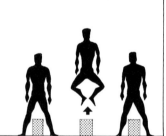

6. In the swimming pool, using a float for your arms, swim with leg kicks only. Then walk forwards, sideways and backwards in the shallow end. Gradually increase speed to run in the water. Build up the time in the water, or the distance of each run.

7. On a mini-trampoline, jog on the spot, then bounce on both legs together, then hop on one leg, building up the time exercising.

8. On a wobble board, balance on one leg, and time how long you can stand perfectly still. Then balance on the board, and bend and straighten your knee, trying to build up to twenty movements on each leg.

9. Run in a straight line, forwards, then sideways and backwards. Jog at first, then build up speed or distance.

10. Hop in a straight line, forwards, then sideways and backwards, building up the number of hops.

11. Kick a ball, straight against a wall. Gradually increase your distance from the wall. Progress to kicking with either leg; running and kicking; then running with the ball and dodging an opponent.

12. Run and turn. Sprint fast, and make sudden changes of direction, preferably with a partner calling out which way you should turn. Alternatively, do shuttle runs, sprinting forwards, touching the ground or bending to simulate the stroke for a racket sport, then turning to run back to the starting point. Do timed intervals or measure your distance, and gradually increase the work.

5 How the Knees are Formed

Three bones make up the knee joint: the thigh-bone (femur), shin-bone (tibia), and the knee-cap (patella). The main part of the knee, which takes your body-weight directly, is formed between the lower end of the thigh-bone and the top of the shin-bone and is technically termed the tibiofemoral joint. The end of the thigh-bone consists of two rounded knuckles, called condyles, which form an enlarged bony area. The condyles are roughly shaped to conform with the flat, elliptical surfaces on

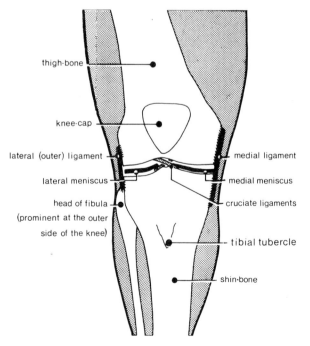

BASIC KNEE STRUCTURE
right knee seen from the front

thigh-bone

knee-cap

lateral (outer) ligament

lateral meniscus

head of fibula
(prominent at the outer
side of the knee)

medial ligament

medial meniscus

cruciate ligaments

tibial tubercle

shin-bone

top of the shin-bone. The area of thigh-bone enclosed within the knee joint is greater than the receiving surface of the shin-bone. There is a natural gap between the two bones, which is filled with fluid. The joint surfaces of the two bones are matched, but they are not perfectly congruent.

The knee-cap and the thigh-bone form a separate, but functionally connected, joint within the knee joint complex, called the patellofemoral joint. The knee-cap is a loose bone, supported in the lower end of the quadriceps muscle group on the front of the thigh. It serves as a kind of pulley between the bulky thigh muscles and their narrow tendon, which links the pointed end of the knee-cap to the bump of the tibial tubercle at the top of the front of the shin. The knee-cap rides over the front of the thigh-bone condyles when you move your knee. Its undersurface is shaped to conform to the contours of the condyles, but a fluid-filled gap separates the knee-cap from the thigh-bone. The patellofemoral joint is not a weight-bearing joint, as it does not transmit any direct loading between your trunk and your feet, but it automatically takes part in any knee movements.

Just below the outer part of the knee is a separate joint which binds the top of the outer leg bone (fibula) to the shin-bone. This is called the superior tibiofibular joint. It is not directly connected to the knee joint, but is indirectly affected by knee movements, especially when you bend and twist your knee.

You can feel many of the knee's bones with your hands. The tibial tubercle is a prominent bump at the top of the front of the shin. To either side of the tubercle, you can feel the horizontal ridge of bone which marks the top of the shin-bone. Just above the tibial tubercle, you can feel the pointed tip of the knee-cap. With your knee straight and relaxed, you can move the knee-cap around freely with your fingers. With your knee bent, you can feel the contours of the thigh-bone condyles in the hollows on either side of the knee-cap. At the side of the knee, you can feel the bump which marks the top of the fibula. This stands out more clearly if you bend your knee, when you can trace the bone by feeling where the cord-like hamstring tendon joins onto it.

44. How the Knees are Formed

Like the other moving joints in the body, the knee is enclosed
in its joint capsule, which is like a covering sack over the bones
forming the joint. The capsule binds round the ends of the
shin-bone and the thigh-bone, but does not cover the knee-cap
or the area of thigh-bone immediately above it, as it is attached
to the sides of the knee-cap.

Parts of the capsule are specially thickened to protect the
knee against abnormal movements, and these thickenings are
called ligaments. Of these ligaments outside the knee joint, the
strongest is the medial ligament, so called because it runs in a
band some six inches long down the inner (medial) edge of
your knee, from thigh-bone to shin-bone. The other technical
name for this ligament is the tibial collateral ligament. On the
other side of the knee, the outer (lateral) ligament is a smaller
band linking the outside of the thigh-bone to the top of the
fibula. Therefore its technical name is the fibular collateral
ligament. The back of the knee is protected by weaker ligaments which cross the back of the joint.

Right in the middle of the knee, there are two very strong
ligaments which bind the knee internally, and are therefore
quite separate from the outer joint capsule. They link the
centre of the thigh-bone to the shin-bone, and are called the
cruciate ligaments, because they form a cross shape where they
pass each other.

The knee-cap joint does not have stabilizing ligaments as
such, although the fibres of the quadriceps muscle which hold
the knee-cap form bonding tissues which blend with the knee's
joint capsule. Confusingly, the tendon which joins the quadriceps muscle to the shin-bone is sometimes called the patellar
ligament, because it acts as a binding tissue between the point
of the knee-cap and the tibial tubercle, but it is functionally a
tendon.

The tibiofibular joint just below the knee is bound together
by a very strong ligament which lies between the shin-bone
and the fibula.

All the ligaments have a specific protective purpose. The
medial and lateral ligaments prevent the knee from moving
sideways. The cruciate ligaments limit any gliding, shearing
and twisting movements between the shin-bone and the thigh-

bone. The ligaments are helped in their protective role by the various muscles and tendons which cross the joint vertically or diagonally on all sides. When the muscles and tendons are not actively contracting to move the knee, they too act to restrict its movements.

THE BUFFERING AND LUBRICATING STRUCTURES OF THE KNEE

The bone surfaces which move within the knee are all covered with cartilage, which is a special type of bone covering. This type of cartilage is a functional part of the bone structure, and is called articular cartilage. It covers the condyles of the thigh-bone, the top of the shin-bone, the back of the knee-cap and the area between the thigh-bone condyles facing the knee-cap. It is not the same as the 'cartilages' made familiar by famous footballers with 'cartilage trouble' through knee injuries.

Those cartilages are soft buffering pads which lie between the thigh-bone and the shin-bone. Because of their crescent shape, they are called semilunar cartilages, or menisci. There are two semilunar cartilages in the knee, lying on either side of the top of the shin-bone. They are attached to the shin-bone by special ligaments which bind the edges of the cartilages to the bone. They are linked to each other at their front edges by a ligament which runs across the top of the shin-bone. The outer cartilage (lateral meniscus) is attached to the cruciate ligament at the front of the knee (anterior cruciate ligament), and it may also be attached to the posterior cruciate ligament at the back of the knee, but it is otherwise relatively free-lying. By contrast, the inner cartilage (medial meniscus) is firmly attached to the knee joint capsule along the whole of its outer edge, and it is also bonded onto the medial ligament.

The knee is lubricated by synovial fluid, like the other moving joints in the body. This fluid is produced by the synovial membrane which lines the joint capsule at the front, sides and back of the knee. The membrane also extends above the knee-cap, where there is no capsule covering, forming a fluid-filled pouch, or bursa, which reaches about two inches above the knee-cap when the knee is straight.

Other, generally smaller bursae lie on all sides of the knee. These are self-contained fluid-filled sacs or pouches, separate from the fluid-forming synovial membrane. They provide cushioning, and, more importantly, friction-free movement between moving parts which would otherwise rub on each other, for instance where a tendon runs over another tendon or bone.

THE MUSCLES AND TENDONS WHICH MOVE THE KNEE

The knee is not a simple hinge-joint. Technically the main knee joint is termed a condylar joint, and it has two degrees of freedom of movement. Besides bending and straightening, it can also twist, or rotate. Some rotatory movement happens automatically when you bend and straighten your knee. As you bend, the shin-bone turns inwards slightly, relative to the thigh-bone; as you straighten, the shin-bone rotates outwards. When your knee is held bent, you can rotate your knee actively and voluntarily. For instance, you can sit with your knees bent, feet on the floor, and bring your toes together, keeping your heels still, by twisting your knees.

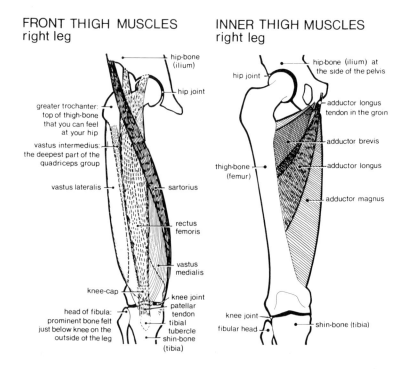

FRONT THIGH MUSCLES
right leg

- hip-bone (ilium)
- hip joint
- greater trochanter: top of thigh-bone that you can feel at your hip
- vastus intermedius: the deepest part of the quadriceps group
- vastus lateralis
- sartorius
- rectus femoris
- vastus medialis
- knee-cap
- head of fibula: prominent bone felt just below knee on the outside of the leg
- knee joint
- patellar tendon
- tibial tubercle
- shin-bone (tibia)

INNER THIGH MUSCLES
right leg

- hip joint
- hip-bone (ilium) at the side of the pelvis
- adductor longus tendon in the groin
- adductor brevis
- thigh-bone (femur)
- adductor longus
- adductor magnus
- knee joint
- fibular head
- shin-bone (tibia)

The knee's movements are governed by the muscles and tendons which cross the joint on each side. The quadriceps muscles lie over the front of the joint, linking the knee-cap to the shin-bone through their attachment tendon, the patellar tendon. The quadriceps work to straighten the knee against gravity or a resistance. The inner quadriceps muscle, vastus medialis, also has a special role in 'locking out' the knee when it is fully straight. You can see the small bulge of vastus medialis just above the inner edge of the knee-cap, when you straighten your knee as hard as you can. When the knee is straight, but relaxed, your quadriceps muscles can pull the knee-cap upwards, in a twitching movement.

Besides the quadriceps, a strong band down the outer side of your thigh and knee can help to straighten the joint. This is the iliotibial tract, which links the side of your seat muscles to the outer side of the top of your shin-bone. It stands out as a firm band when you straighten your knee hard. The popliteus muscle lies across the back of the knee, linking the outer knuckle on the thigh-bone with the upper end of the shin-bone. It helps to bend the knee, especially when the joint is 'unlocked' from the fully straightened position.

HAMSTRING MUSCLES
on back of right thigh

CALF MUSCLES
on back of right leg

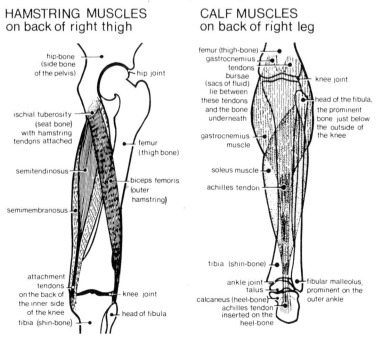

48. How the Knees are Formed

The hamstring tendons lie over the back of the knee, so they can bend the knee against gravity or a resistance. The bulky calf muscle (gastrocnemius) also extends over the back of the knee, so it can help the bending movement when necessary. You can feel the hamstring tendons behind the knee if you sit with your knee bent and press your heel gently backwards into the floor. With your hand behind your knee, you can feel the cords of the hamstring tendons standing out at the back of your thigh.

The muscles at the sides of the knee perform the knee's twisting movements. The outer hamstring tendon (biceps femoris) turns your foot outwards from the knee. The inner hamstrings (semitendinosus and semimembranosus) turn your foot inwards, helped by the muscles which curve round the inner side of the joint, which have the descriptive name of 'goose's foot' (pes anserinus).

Apart from its independent twitching movement, the knee-cap is moved automatically when the knee moves. The tibiofibular joint below the knee moves very slightly when the knee works, but it has no independent movement at all, so you cannot move this joint at will.

ILIOTIBIAL TRACT ON THE OUTER SIDE OF THE RIGHT THIGH

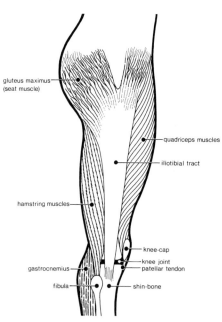

gluteus maximus (seat muscle)

quadriceps muscles

iliotibial tract

hamstring muscles

knee-cap

knee joint

patellar tendon

gastrocnemius

fibula

shin-bone

HOW THE KNEE GROWS

The basic structure of the knee, as the joint between the bottom of the thigh-bone and the top of the shin-bone, is present from the day a child is born. Logically, the structural details develop as the child grows up. A child's bones are relatively pliable, and are formed in parts, which gradually grow together, hardening into each single bone when the bone reaches its final shape and size. In the child's knee, the ends of the thigh-bone and the shin-bone are separated from the main shafts of their respective bones by a disc of growth cartilage, called the epiphyseal plate. The bone ends complete their growth and fuse onto their shafts by about the age of sixteen in girls, and eighteen in boys. The tibial tubercle starts to grow from the front of the growing part of the shin-bone at about the age of ten, and fuses onto the shaft of the bone at about fifteen in girls, seventeen in boys. The knee-cap only starts to grow when a child is about three, but its separate parts quickly fuse together into a single bone.

As the bones grow, so the soft tissues around them have to develop, especially the muscles and tendons. In teenagers going through the phase of puberty, muscle growth is accompanied by adjustments in the fat cover lying between the muscles and the skin. Girls gain fat, especially over the thighs, seat and abdomen. This gives them the smooth rounded contours of maturity. Boys lose their fat cover, so that their muscles gradually become more clearly defined as they gain size and strength.

The age at which puberty arrives varies with the individual. Growth spurts, when the bones go through a phase of very rapid development, may happen at any time up to the phase of final fusion. During a growth spurt, the teenager's muscles may seem relatively tight and weak, until they catch up with the bone development. The way in which the muscles develop is determined partly through heredity, partly through diet, and partly through the patterns of normal use which establish relative strength and flexibility in the muscle groups controlling the knees.

6 What Makes Knees Hurt

These can happen to the knee in two ways: through trauma or overuse.

Traumatic injuries can also be classified as extrinsic injuries, because they always have an external, recognisable cause. A traumatic injury occurs when an accident causes abnormal stress to the knee, resulting in damage. The injury may be only slight, involving no more than a minor strain, or it may be major, including bone breakage or rupture of ligaments or tendons. Occasionally, there is a delayed reaction, and the signs of the damage only become noticeable some time after the accident. More often, the symptoms, which are usually varying degrees of pain, swelling and disability, follow immediately or quickly, and are unmistakably related to the accident.

Accidents can happen to anyone at any time. The knee is vulnerable to twisting and shearing strains, and injuries through over-compression and over-stretching. It can be hurt when the joint is straight, but it is especially at risk when it is bent. A sudden turn while walking can be enough to injure the knee; a fall down steps can hurt the knee badly. An awkward landing from a jump can jar the joint, for instance when a lorry or bus driver jumps down from the cab. Workers who spend a lot of time crouching, squatting or kneeling, like gardeners, electricians and carpet-layers, can hurt their knees through just slightly awkward movements. Energetic dances like the Charleston, Twist and Limbo stress the knees to their limits, so that slight over-balancing can cause injury. Sports which carry a high risk of knee trauma through twisting, jarring or shearing include rugby, American football, soccer, ice and field hockey, downhill ski-ing, and weightlifting.

Overuse injuries can be called intrinsic injuries, because they usually come on without an obvious cause. They are often surreptitious, starting with no more than a slight ache, which gradually gets worse if the activity that causes the reaction is continued. Apart from the increasing pain, there is usually little else to show for the injury in terms of swelling and disability, unless the problem is allowed to develop to a severe stage.

Overuse injuries can occur at any age, and although they seem to happen without a cause, in fact they are often due to various predisposing factors. Mechanical imbalance in the muscles controlling the knee can be one of these factors. For instance, there may be relative weakness of the vastus medialis muscle in relation to the rest of the quadriceps muscle group; or the hamstring muscles may be tight or weak compared to the quadriceps group. Fatigue and stiffness are other factors which can affect the knee's efficiency. Growth and ageing processes can make a person more vulnerable to overuse syndromes. Painful osteoarthritis, or wear-and-tear, can be the result of cumulative minute damage through a lifetime's use of the joint, or it can come on as the delayed result of an injury which happened years previously. In childhood and adolescence the knee's bones are prone to gradual damage in their growth and fusion phases, while in old age the bones may be weakened by a condition called senile osteoporosis. Inactivity can weaken the bones in people of any age who have been immobilised for a long time, for instance by spending months in bed through illness: this is called disuse osteoporosis. In women, the bones become more vulnerable at the menopause, because of the reduction of the female hormone, oestrogen. It is thought that similar bone weakening may happen in younger women who stop having periods through anorexia or hard exercise. Diet may play a part in bone and muscle overuse injury problems, if the food intake is deficient in vital ingredients like minerals, or if the fluid intake is inadequate.

Overuse injuries are typically associated with activities and sports which involve repetitive movements, like walking, running, cycling and swimming. A slight change in the normal pattern of movement can bring on pain through altered stresses, for instance through wearing different shoes, or walking or running on camber or hilly ground. An increase in the amount of any repetitive activity can cause injury, like an unusually long walk or stepped-up training for running, cycling or swimming. The category of overuse injuries also includes problems due to disuse and misuse. Sitting with the knees bent for long periods undermines vastus medialis, creating muscular imbalance in the quadriceps muscle group, and setting the scene for knee-cap pain. Sitting with the knees twisted at awkward angles places abnormal stress on the ligaments which limit the knees' twisting movements. Inactivity, as in lying down or sitting still for long periods, hinders the normal lubrication of the knees and makes them stiff. Driving a car or van with insufficient leg room prevents full extension at the knees, causing vastus medialis weakness and quadriceps imbalance. Crouching, squatting or kneeling for long periods can cause similar problems.

REFERRED PAIN

This can affect the knee, causing pain which seems to be in the knee itself, but which in fact stems from somewhere else in the body, usually the hip or back. This type of pain is often described as a 'pinched nerve', because the pain is transmitted through a nerve pathway from the source where the nerve is being irritated. The pain may be localised exactly in the knee, or there may be a line of pain travelling up the thigh towards the pain source. The pain may seem to pass along the front, side or back of the thigh, according to which part of the back or hip it stems from.

Sometimes knee problems are complicated by referred pain appearing on top of a simple injury to the knee. Diagnosis and treatment have to be directed at both causes of the pain in the knee. In children, it is particularly important to obtain an accurate diagnosis of whether knee pain is caused by localised injury, referred pain, or both, as one important cause of a child's knee pain can be a potentially serious hip problem called a slipped epiphysis.

Pain referred to the knee usually seems arbitrary, coming on with no recognisable pattern, but close analysis often shows that the pain occurs in relation to certain postures or movements involving the hip or back. Another indication that the pain might be referred can be odd sensations of tingling or numbness occurring in the pathway of the affected nerve, along the thigh or round the knee. These sensations sometimes alternate with the pain felt, or occasionally replace it.

DISEASES

Various kinds can cause knee pain which, like referred pain, seems exactly like the pain of an injury. Inflammatory conditions like rheumatoid arthritis or gout can cause sudden, often severe, pain in the knee. Usually the affected joint swells up quickly and feels hot and uncomfortable. It may look reddened and the skin may seem shiny. There are many different inflammatory conditions which can cause joint pain. Psoriatic arthritis is an example in which the joint swelling and pain tend to accompany flare-ups in the skin condition, psoriasis. Many of these conditions affect several different joints in the body, either at different times, or together. If only one joint is affected, with no apparent involvement of any other joints, the condition is usually called a monarticular arthritis. Many of the inflammatory conditions, like rheumatoid arthritis, tend to run in families. Some, like gout, may seem to be triggered or affected by changes in diet, to richer or fattier foods, or an increase in alcohol intake, especially of the 'heavier' drinks like sherry, port or red wine. Infection can cause sudden pain or swelling in the knee, usually accompanied by a burning feeling. A bone tumour close to the knee usually causes gradual pain and swelling, giving almost exactly the same symptoms at first as an overuse injury.

Fortunately, serious conditions of this kind are relatively rare. But the possibility that they may occur makes it essential to have an accurate diagnosis of the knee problem, before embarking on what might be inappropriate treatment. Sometimes diagnosis is complicated because the medical condition happens to a sportsman, or to someone who has also suffered an accident or injury involving the knee. However, it is usually possible to work out cause and effect, if an accurate picture of how the pain came on, and how it behaves, is presented to the doctor or specialist.

7 How Specialists Identify Knee Problems

An accurate description of what has happened in any knee problem is crucial to establishing exactly what is wrong. Technically, the description of an injury, pain or other symptoms is called the history of the problem, because it involves a detailed factual explanation of the sequence of events relating to it. When a doctor or surgeon examines an injured knee, a clear history is the first step towards the correct diagnosis. Conversely, a muddled description can seriously confuse matters. If a chartered physiotherapist or physical therapist is misled by a garbled history when assessing a problem knee, the wrong type of treatment may be applied. All practitioners establish the history of a problem by asking questions. They usually write down the information they are given, for reference. It helps if you have prepared the answers to the possible questions, before your knee is examined. Writing down the relevant facts saves time and improves the accuracy of your account. The information needed covers the problem directly first, but most practitioners also require some background facts. The questions may cover some or all of the following points, depending on circumstances.

• Are both knees troubling you, or just one? What happened to your problem knee(s)? If you suffered an injury, was the joint twisted, jarred or wrenched; was your weight on the injured leg; was any external force applied? If there was no distinct injury, what made you aware something was wrong, and what exactly were you doing at the time you first noticed it?

• When did the injury happen, or when did you first notice the symptoms? Try to note down the date, and the time of day.

- Is there pain in the problem knee(s)? If there is, whereabouts in the joint(s) do you feel the pain? Does the pain get worse on certain movements; during the night; and/or at rest? Is it severe, or only an ache? Is the pain progressively getting worse? Does anything relieve it? If both knees hurt, did they become painful at the same time, or separately?

- Is there stiffness in the knee(s)? If so, did the stiffness come on suddenly or gradually? Which movements are limited? Are any movements completely blocked? Is the stiffness becoming more noticeable?

- Is there swelling in the knee(s)? If so, did the swelling appear suddenly or slowly? Has it increased, decreased or remained the same since it first appeared? If both knees are swollen, did they swell up at the same time, or separately?

- Have you noticed warmth or redness in the knee(s)?

- Have you felt numbness or tingling in the knee(s)?

- Is there a 'clicking' sound in the knee(s)? If so, whereabouts in the joint do you feel the click, and which movements cause it?

- Is there a 'catching' feeling in the knee(s)? If so, which movements cause it?

- Have you felt the knee(s) lock? If so, has the joint become completely stuck, so that you can only free it by twisting the knee in a certain way with your hands? Or is it blocked from certain movements by pain alone?

- Have you felt the knee(s) give way? If so, have you fallen over, or is there just a momentary giving sensation?

- Had you changed your normal routine when, or immediately before, your knee problem started? You should note any unusual activities, like extended periods digging or weeding in the garden, or crouching under the car doing repairs. The sports player should record any changes of technique or training, or any specially long sessions playing, practising or competing.

- Had you changed your diet, eaten any food you were not used to, drunk unusual soft or alcoholic drinks, or drunk an excessive amount of alcohol immediately before your knee problem started?

• Have you had any notable illnesses before or since having knee problems?

• Does anyone in your family suffer from an inflammatory condition like rheumatoid arthritis?

• Had you injured this knee or experienced problems in it before? The adult should try particularly to remember any teenage pains in the joint.

• Have you had back or hip problems?

• Had there been any muscle or joint problems in the same leg before the knee problem started? Had there been any problems with the other leg?

• What kind of shoes were you wearing when the knee injury happened or the problem came on? Were they new, or very worn down? (If the shoes might have contributed to the problem, they should be brought in for inspection.)

FROM THE ASSESSMENT

Having listened to the story of the knee problem, the practitioner usually goes on to look at the injured joint(s). If only one knee is affected, comparison is made with the uninjured knee in terms of appearance and function. The visual examination is followed by tests to show up functional weaknesses in the various knee structures. Your description provides the practitioner with the symptoms of the problem, that is the sensations which have made you aware that something is wrong. The physical examination and tests provide facts which are technically called 'clinical signs'. The signs and symptoms together may be enough evidence for the doctor or surgeon to reach a conclusion, and provide a diagnosis. If there is doubt about the nature of the problem, the next stage in the examining process is the internal checks, or investigations, like blood tests and X-rays. Once the diagnosis has been reached, you may be referred to a practitioner like a chartered physiotherapist or physical therapist for treatment, and your knee will be examined and assessed again. This may seem like duplication, but the aim of the assessment is different, as the physiotherapist needs to establish the priorities of treatment for your individual problem.

The physical assessment may take place in the family doctor's surgery, the casualty department, the specialist's consulting room, the sports clinic, or the physiotherapy department or treatment room. If your visit is by appointment, rather than an emergency, try to remember that you will need to reveal both legs to the practitioner, so clothing that is easy to remove is an advantage. You may be asked, or prefer, to wear shorts for the examination: if not, modest underwear is in order. If you have been using knee supports or protective padding of any kind, you should bring them with you for the practitioner to see. Sports players should always bring in all pairs of sports shoes in current use, in case they are significant in the knee problem.

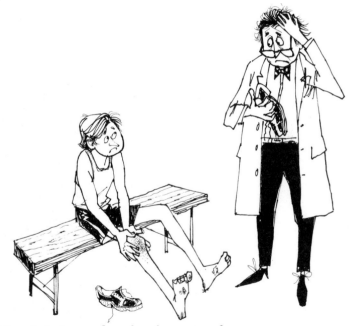

Knee injuries can be related to sports shoes

The order in which the assessment is done, and the particular tests which are performed, vary according to the practitioner and the problem. The examination usually starts with the visual check, as the practitioner looks for outward signs of damage, and compares both knees. Simple functional tests to find out how many of its normal movements the knee can perform may follow. You may be asked to sit up on a couch, so that your feet are supported, and bend and straighten your knees one at a time or both together. The angle to which each knee can bend may be measured with a kind of protractor called a goniometer. If your knee is very swollen, painful and difficult to move, you are unlikely to be asked to perform any movements standing with your body-weight over it. If your problem is only slight, you may be asked to stand up and squat down; balance on your injured leg and bend the knee; run-on-the-spot; hop in all directions; and squat-walk (crouch down and walk on fully bent knees).

The examination usually includes tests to show how well the muscles controlling the knee are working. To test vastus medialis, the 'locking-out' muscle which straightens the knee, you may be asked to stand and twitch your knee-cap by tightening your thigh muscles slightly: if vastus medialis is very weak, you may be unable to do this. You may then be

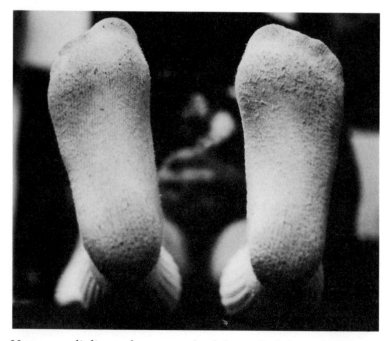

Vastus medialis weakness: one heel drops slightly as the knee fails to hold itself fully straight

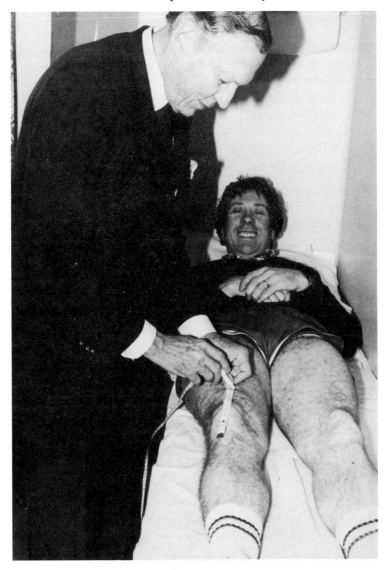

Measuring the thigh muscles

asked to flicker the knee-cap by tightening the thigh muscles rapidly. If this is difficult, the co-ordinated action of vastus medialis has been undermined. Sitting on the couch with your legs straight in front of you, you may be asked to tighten your thigh muscles to straighten your knees as hard as you can, while you pull your toes towards you back from the ankles, so that, if possible, your heels lift away from the couch. Keeping you sitting on the couch, the practitioner may pull your relaxed leg as straight as it will go, and then ask if you can hold your knee fully straight while he releases his hold on your heel: if your foot drops down when he lets go, vastus medialis is weak. Finally, while you are still sitting on the couch, the practitioner may place a support under your knee to bend it, and then test how well you can straighten each knee in turn against the pressure of his hand pushing down over the front of your ankles. More generalised tests for the other knee muscles involve checking their power by making them work against the resistance of the practitioner's hand. You are asked to bend the knee, straighten it from bent, lift the leg straight up backwards and sideways, while the practitioner opposes each movement. Most of these tests are done on the couch, and you may have to turn onto your stomach and each side in turn. The simplest muscle test is to measure their girth with a tape. The most sophisticated way of testing knee muscle power is by using computerised measuring systems, for example the Kin Com or Cybex II.

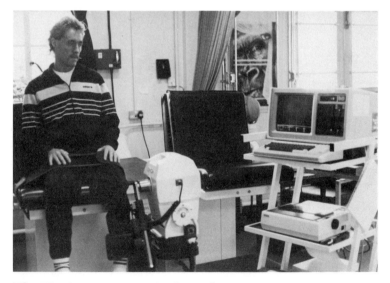

The Kin Com, computerised muscle measuring equipment (photo courtesy the Royal National Orthopaedic Hospital, Stanmore)

Palpation is the technical term for feeling the joint with the hands. It is an important part of the physical examination, showing up sore spots, unusual thickening and abnormal motion. The practitioner presses over the various structures of the knee that can be felt through the skin, while you sit on the couch. Your knee may be bent or slightly twisted, to bring specific parts of the structures under the practitioner's hand. You may be sitting up or lying on your back while the front and sides of the knee are examined, while the back of the knee is usually checked with you lying on your stomach. Most of the knee's outer structures can be felt with the hands, including the inner (medial) and outer (lateral) ligaments, the iliotibial tract, the outer surface of the knee-cap, and the patellar tendon. Some of the knee's bone surfaces can be felt through the skin as well.

Passive movement tests are used to check for pain or limited function in the knee's structures, and they can show up damage in the innermost structures of the knee, such as the cruciate ligaments, which cannot be felt from the outside. These tests involve twisting or bending the knee in such a way as to put pressure or stress on the structures being tested. For instance, pulling the shin-bone outwards on the thigh-bone so that the knee bends inwards (valgus stress) shows whether the inner side (medial) ligament is holding correctly. Pulling the shin-bone the other way reveals any looseness in the outer side (lateral) ligament. In the Lachman test for the anterior cruciate ligament, the practitioner holds the knee slightly bent and pulls the top of the shin-bone gently forwards: if the ligament is torn or over-stretched, the shin-bone glides forwards further than normal in relation to the thigh-bone. In the anterior drawer test for the anterior cruciate ligament, you sit on the couch with your knee bent to a right angle, and the practitioner blocks your foot, usually by sitting on it; he pulls the top of your shin-bone gently forwards from behind with his hands, to see if there is abnormal forward gliding of the shin-bone relative to the thigh-bone. The posterior drawer test shows damage to the posterior cruciate ligament, if pushing the shin-bone backwards from the same position makes the shin drop back too far in relation to the thigh-bone. Another test for the anterior cruciate ligament is the pivot shift or jerk test, in which the practitioner holds the heel, twists the shin-bone inwards and gently bends and straightens the knee, while applying

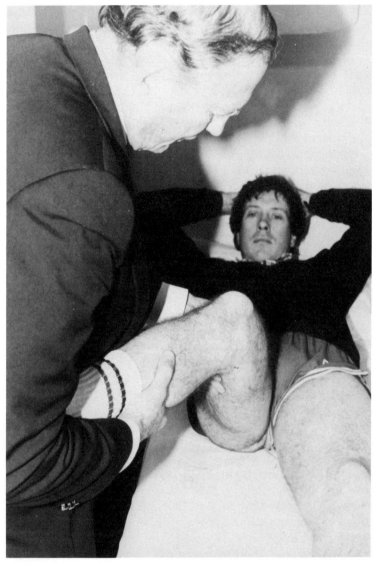

Testing the medial (inner side) ligament

upward pressure against the heel: if the anterior cruciate is not
holding properly, the outer side of the knee seems to be out of
place when the knee is slightly bent, but the shin-bone drops
back into place with a jump as the knee is bent further. There
are also many tests for cartilage tears. One of the most com-

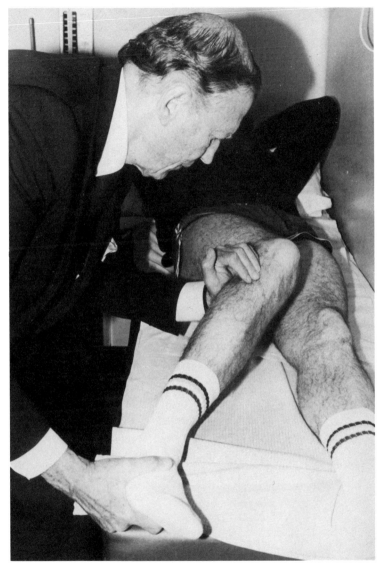

Lateral pivot shift test

monly used is McMurray's test, in which you lie on your back on the couch, and the practitioner feels the knee with one hand, using the other to hold the foot or ankle and twist the joint while the knee is gently bent: at a certain point, the knee may give a 'clunk', or lock, indicating that the cartilage is torn.

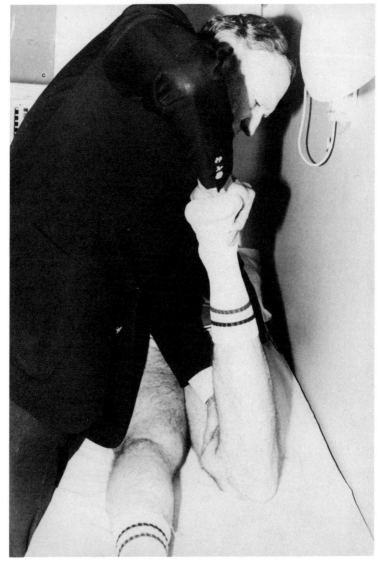

The Apley grind test for cartilage tear

Another cartilage test is the grind test, in which you lie on your stomach, and the practitioner bends your knee while holding your foot, presses down against your knee through your heel, and twists the shin-bone to either side: this may catch a torn cartilage, causing pain and sometimes a click.

THROUGH INVESTIGATIONS

In many cases of knee injury, the history and physical assessment provide sufficient basis for so-called conservative, or non-invasive treatment, such as physiotherapy techniques. Investigations become necessary when the doctor or surgeon is in doubt abut the diagnosis, or when confirmation of the diagnosis is needed before proceeding to more invasive, or drastic, treatment, like an operation. The investigations ordered by the doctor depend on the particular problem affecting the knee, and the doctor's suspicions as to what might be wrong. Many investigations may be done to prove a diagnosis by excluding the other possible causes of a problem.

If the problem knee is badly swollen, the doctor may drain off, or aspirate, the excess fluid, partly to make the knee more comfortable, but also in order to have the fluid analysed in the laboratory, if there is any suspicion of an infection or some disease in the joint.

Biopsy is the analysis of tissues taken from the body, and it may be used to check for infection or disease in small pieces of synovial tissue, articular cartilage or bone removed during surgery.

Blood tests may be ordered to identify diseases, or inflammatory conditions affecting the joint.

X-rays show bone defects, injuries or abnormalities, including unusually large or small gaps between the knee-bones. They may be taken with the knee straight or bent, from the front, or from either side. Stress X-rays are taken with pressure applied against the knee, as in the passive movement tests, to show if a ligament is not holding properly. X-rays are normally taken by radiographers, and read, or interpreted, by doctors, surgeons or radiologists. Radiologists are doctors specially trained in X-ray interpretation, and they are normally asked for an opinion on the diagnosis, without being involved in eventual treatment.

Arthrograms are special X-rays taken after dye has been injected into the knee joint. They show up tears or defects in the soft tissues, like the cartilages.

Bone scans are images gained by injecting radioactive material (radioisotopes) into the blood stream, and filming the reaction round the joint some time later. The bone scan, in conjunction with other confirming tests, shows up infections, inflammatory diseases, and any kind of bone problem, including the stress fracture which is usually 'invisible' on normal X-rays. The 'CAT scan', properly termed the computerised axial tomogram, uses computers to create layered X-ray images of the leg, as though slices were cut directly through it. This can show accurately any kind of damage affecting the shape of the bones or soft tissues.

Arthroscopy is a relatively minor operation, in which the surgeon inserts a kind of periscope into the knee. The arthroscope has a light and a magnifying glass on its tip, so the surgeon can manoeuvre it to see right round the joint. Although you normally have to have a general anaesthetic for arthroscopy, the instrument is inserted through a tiny hole, so recovery from the operation is extremely quick. One advantage of arthroscopy is that surgery such as the removal of the

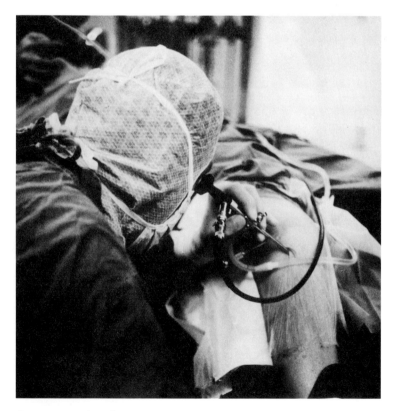

Surgeon and arthroscope

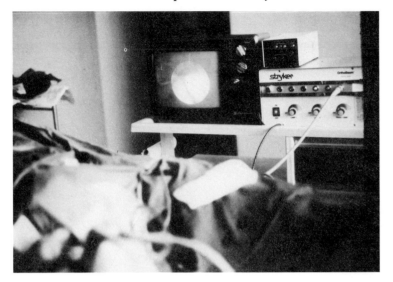

A camera on the arthroscope gives the surgeon an enlarged television picture of the inside of the knee

torn parts of a cartilage, can often be performed through the arthroscope, eliminating the need to cut the knee open with a scar. Therefore arthroscopy has helped to make both the diagnosis and the treatment of certain knee injuries much more rapid.

8 How to Cope with Knee Problems

Everyone, and especially anyone involved in sport, should do a standard first-aid course, in order to know exactly what to do when an accident happens. (That said, it is as important to know what not to do, in an emergency.) Assessing priorities quickly is essential to effective first-aid care. When traumatic accidents happen to the knee, some of the following actions will probably need to be taken:

• Stop any bleeding. A small cut can be simply washed under the tap, dried with a clean towel or swab, and covered with sticking plaster. A slit cut, if clean, can be effectively held together with butterfly plasters (tiny strips of plasters which bind across the cut just as stitches would). A large wound must be staunched by holding a clean dressing, or any relatively clean material, over the wound until the bleeding stops. If the bleeding is heavy, and the dressing becomes soaked, it may be necessary to press further dressings over the original one, which should not be removed until the bleeding has stopped or medical help arrives. Even if it is not possible to clean the wound first, the priority is to cover the wound to stop the bleeding. Excessive bleeding can lead to clinical shock, a state in which the body's vital systems stop receiving enough oxygen, which can result in death, in the worst of cases. Direct pressure over the wound is the best way to stop the bleeding. Tourniquets which stop the blood flow into the area through pressure over the supplying arteries can cause damage to otherwise unaffected areas. Burns and grazes can be treated similarly to wounds, with fresh water cleansing, and possibly a dry dressing covering.

• Apply ice for any bruising or swelling. The technical term for applying ice to an injury is cryotherapy. Ice should be applied immediately to limit internal bleeding, bruising or swelling. It also helps to relieve pain. Ice cubes can be rubbed gently over the knee; or they can be laid in a wet towel and wrapped round the knee. An ice pack must be applied with due care for the skin, either over a damp towel, or on skin that has been protected using olive or baby oil. Chemical ice applications, such as cold-wrap bandages or chemical ice packs, can be used, but the manufacturer's directions must be followed carefully. The ice can be applied for up to twenty minutes or even longer, but should be taken off if the victim suffers discomfort from it. Even four minutes of ice application, done immediately, can be helpful, and sometimes ice is better tolerated if it is applied for short spells only, and then repeated at half-hourly or hourly intervals. If the ice is applied for longer periods, it should be re-applied every two hours or so, until the victim receives medical help. If there is any sign of the skin becoming sore, the ice applications should be stopped. Ice may also be needed in later phases of the knee injury, if there is persistent swelling.

• Bandage the joint. To alleviate the pain, control any swelling, and protect the knee from harmful movements, a firm bandage should be applied. For a relatively minor injury, the bandage should extend from roughly five inches below the knee to five inches above it. For more serious damage, the bandage should be started at ankle level, and reach up almost to the groin. A single or double tubular (stocking) bandage may be sufficient. For firmer support, the leg can be encased in a wadding of cotton wool, covered by a crepe bandage. If even greater support is needed to keep the knee comfortable, more layers of the cotton wool and bandage can be applied. An inflatable splint for the whole leg, carefully applied, can be an alternative means of immobilising the knee, but it must not be over-inflated, and the victim should be shown how to reduce the pressure, if the splint starts to feel tight. In most cases, the injured knee is straightened gently, and then bandaged straight. If the knee is locked, or too painful to straighten, wadding is placed behind the knee, and it is bandaged in the bent position.

• Splint the leg, if there is an obvious bone break, and the casualty has to wait, or be moved, before professional help arrives. Apart from being encased in an inflatable splint, the injured leg can be tied with bandages or other material to a long stick, or to the other leg, with soft padding between the leg and its support. In most cases, the leg is splinted with the knee held straight, but if this is too uncomfortable, the knee can rest on soft material in the bent position, and the splint can be tied along the back of the leg.

• Check the circulation. Whenever a bandage or splint has been applied, the circulation of the injured leg must be checked at five- or ten-minute intervals, in case the bandaging is too tight, or has become restrictive through increasing swelling in the injured knee. The circulation can be checked by feeling whether the pulse on the top of the foot is still beating. More simply, if the nail on the big toe is squeezed, it turns white, and should turn pink again immediately. If the pulse has disappeared, or the toe-nail stays white for longer than an instant, the bandaging should be loosened immediately.

• Elevate the leg, to prevent blood and tissue fluid from being pushed into the injured knee and down into the lower leg through the pressure of gravity. Whether the casualty sits up or lies down, the injured leg should be supported, preferably on soft material, so that the foot is held above the level of the hip.

• Encourage muscle maintenance. Even in the first moments after an injury, once the knee has been made comfortable, the victim should be told to try to work the quadriceps muscles, simply by twitching them very gently, so that the knee-cap moves slightly. Even if this causes pain at first, the effort should be repeated just a few times at ten-minute intervals. If the pain is not too great, the casualty may be able to lift the leg straight up forwards, backwards and sideways. The muscle work must be encouraged because the knee muscles are inhibited immediately when the joint is injured. The vastus medialis muscle wastes particularly rapidly, within about six hours of a knee injury, while the rest of the thigh muscles are badly weakened within 24–36 hours. Starting the static thigh muscle contractions as quickly as possible can save the victim a lot of secondary problems later on.

• Transfer to hospital. An obviously severe injury will probably require ambulance transport to hospital as an emergency, especially if there are broken bones and profuse bleeding. Even if the injury does not seem grossly disabling, a badly swollen knee should also be seen as quickly as possible by a medical specialist. As surgery may be needed, the victim should not be allowed to eat or drink anything, apart from possibly sipping enough water just to moisten the lips. No weight should be taken through the badly injured leg, so if the victim is not carried on a stretcher, he or she should hop, preferably with another person acting as a human crutch.

WHICH SPECIALIST?

The person who has had an accident warranting hospital treatment as a casualty is usually seen in the Accident and Emergency Department by the casualty officer, who may be an accident surgeon or an orthopaedic surgeon. The doctor examining the injury may decide to admit the casualty into the hospital for immediate surgery or immobilisation in bed. The more minor injury may be bandaged or put in a plaster cast, and the casualty sent home. Follow-up treatment is usually arranged, which may consist of review of the injury at intervals by an orthopaedic specialist, or rehabilitation treatment from a chartered physiotherapist.

Away from the emergency situation, the problem of which specialist to see with any given knee condition may seem unnecessarily complicated. In fact, the best starting point is the general practitioner or family doctor. He is a central reference point, with an overall view of his patients' whole medical history. He is therefore well placed to analyse a patient's problem in the context of his total health picture. The general practitioner may be able to treat the knee problem himself. If not, he can decide which type of investigations might be needed, and which specialist the patient should be referred to. The general practitioner may organize investigations like blood tests and X-rays himself, or he may leave the whole process of diagnosis to the specialist.

The orthopaedic surgeon is likely to be consulted for any knee injury or problem involving mechanical cause and effect, which needs specialist analysis, and which might need surgical repair. The orthopaedic surgeon usually practises other types of physical medicine treatments, apart from surgery, notably injections, manipulation and drug therapy. The orthopaedic doctor is a specialist who offers similar physical treatments, but normally does not operate surgically, so he may be consulted if it seems that surgery is not necessary.

If there is no obvious cause for a knee problem, and therefore a possibility that it stems from a disease or an inflammatory condition, such as rheumatoid arthritis or gout, the general practitioner is likely to refer the patient to a rheumatologist, a specialist in joint, bone and soft-tissue problems involving internal mechanisms. The rheumatologist performs investigations to identify the cause of the problem, and then offers appropriate treatment, often involving drug therapy. Rehabilitation and treatment from a chartered physiotherapist may also be recommended for many conditions. The rheumatologist does not normally perform surgical operations, so he refers the patient to an orthopaedic specialist, if surgical repair is to be part of the cure.

The homoeopathic doctor is another medical specialist the general practitioner might refer to for treatment for a non-mechanical injury. Homoeopathy tends to use naturally occurring substances rather than synthetic drugs for cure, and it works on the principle that the body's healing mechanisms are stimulated by very small quantities of substances which produce similar effects to those produced by the particular disease or problem. Qualified homoeopathic doctors may also be qualified as surgeons, so they may be able to offer a variety of solutions to the patient.

Rehabilitation is a necessary part of recovery in many knee problems, and this usually involves care from a qualified paramedic. It may be applied as the main line of treatment following a relatively simple injury; as a follow-up to surgery; in the recovery phase after an infection; or for maintenance and improvement in long-standing (chronic) conditions, disabilities or diseases. The chartered physiotherapist, or physical therapist, is trained in exercise therapy, hydrotherapy (pool exercises), electrotherapy, chest physiotherapy, massage and manipulation. These skills are applied in order to ease pain, improve mobility and strength, and restore physical function. The remedial gymnast is specially trained in exercise therapy to help active recovery. The athletic trainer, in the United States, is specially trained in sports physiotherapy, and therefore can help in the types of injuries incurred in sport. If special splints or supports are needed, the orthotist or occupational therapist may fit and supply them. If the knee problem is related to poor foot function, the podiatrist, a chiropodist specially trained in foot mechanics, makes individually fitted foot supports or orthotics.

The dietician and the nutritionist are relevant practitioners for those knee conditions where excessive weight is aggravating the problem, or where dietary deficiencies might be contributing to the condition.

Beyond the scope of standard ethical medicine, 'alternative medicine' may offer some solutions to knee problems. Osteopaths and chiropractors are specially trained manipulators, and they can be particularly useful when a knee problem is associated with a back condition. A naturopath usually applies treatment based on diet correction and herbal medicines. The acupuncturist is trained in the long-standing art of healing needles. The reflexologist aims to cure pain and malfunctions through healing meridians in the foot. A patient referring to an 'alternative practitioner' may or may not have the approval or recommendation of his general practitioner. If not, simple precautions to take are to check that the practitioner is registered with the appropriate professional body, and possibly to find out if the practitioner is covered by professional indemnity insurance, in case treatment should go wrong.

As there are so many different practitioners who might help a knee condition, it is impossible for the patient to decide which is the correct person to consult, as this involves diagnosing the cause of the problem. The easiest way to make a mistake is to consult a practitioner on the basis that he helped a friend who had 'the same problem'. An even worse mistake is to consult several practitioners independently of each other. The principles of caring for any knee problem, whether traumatic, overuse or inflammatory, include controlling the pain and swelling; protecting the damaged knee by limiting painful weight-bearing and supporting the knee in an appropriate type of bandage, cast or splint; and applying corrective exercise to stabilise the knee and then restore its mobility. If a practitioner seems to be achieving these aims, or can explain why a particular line of treatment will do so, the patient should follow through the treatment, even if progress seems slow. If there is no progress, and no satisfactory explanation of the diagnosis and likely course of the problem, the patient should refer to another practitioner for a further opinion. This should only be done through the central reference point, usually the general practitioner, who can identify the best person to see in the circumstances, and who holds the record of the investigations done and the treatments tried. In this way, haphazard, conflicting, or duplicated investigations and treatments can be avoided.

GETTING ABOUT WITH A KNEE PROBLEM

Unless the problem is severe enough to keep the victim in bed, it is usually necessary to learn how to move around safely without damaging a painful knee. A wheelchair may be needed temporarily in the early stages of recovery, either for convenience, or if it is too difficult to be upright because of a heavy plaster or excessive pain. The injured knee needs to be supported on a padded board, so that it is kept elevated and straight. It is undesirable to sit in the wheelchair for too long at a time, as the victim's back may become very stiff and sore: it should be used purely in order to get around quickly.

At home, it may not always be convenient to use a wheelchair or crutches. It may be possible to hop around, if the knee is well bandaged. Stairs are a problem in this situation: often the easiest way is to go up and down on one's bottom by sitting on the step with the injured leg held clear, and propelling oneself up backwards using the strong leg and the arms, reversing the process to come down forwards. If the leg can take weight, one can walk stiff-legged. Stairs are negotiated one at a time, with the injured leg coming up behind. Going down is easiest sideways, with the injured leg going down first.

Normally crutches are used to protect the knee in the first stages of recovery, immediately after the injury, or when the patient first gets out of bed after surgery. There are two types of crutches, those which reach to just below the armpits, called axillary crutches, and shorter ones, called elbow crutches, which extend up to about the middle of the upper arm. Axillary crutches are usually made of wood, and are likely to be chosen for you if you are tall and heavily built. Elbow crutches are usually metal and lightweight. Crutches are usually adjusted for height by aligning the hand grip with the wrist, while the patient stands upright with hands relaxed down, wearing the shoes that will be used for moving around. Sensible shoes must be worn: they should be flat or low-heeled, with non-slip soles, and they should lace up or fit snugly to the feet. The elbows are held slightly bent, when the patient stands upright holding the crutches. The elbow crutches cradle the upper arm. The axillary crutches must be pressed into the chest: if the patient rests the armpits on the top of the crutches, the arm nerves can be paralysed by the pressure, a condition called crutch-palsy.

If the knee is to be kept completely unloaded, the patient has to hop, using the crutches for support. The crutches are placed forwards and slightly outwards; the patient presses down on the hand grips for support and hops to stand between the crutches; and then repeats the process to move forward. Once the movement is familiar, the patient can hop to land just in front of the crutches, in the 'swing-through gait', which makes crutch walking quicker. Going up stairs with crutches, the patient stands close to the stair, balanced on the crutches, and hops up to the next step by pressing down on the crutches, leaving them on the lower step; then the crutches are brought up and the process repeated. Coming down stairs, the crutches are placed down on the lower step first, and the patient hops down to them, taking care to keep the crutches and the weight-bearing foot well in the centre of the stair. It is much easier to go up and down stairs using one crutch and a bannister rail, using the same pattern of movement as with two crutches.

Crutches become dangerous when the rubber tips are worn down, so these must be checked and replaced when necessary. They become very slippery in wet weather, so care must be taken not to place them too far away from the body, and not to move around too fast. Walking with crutches impedes mobility, so extra time must be allowed when crossing busy roads.

Once the knee is ready to take weight, the crutches can be used to allow a gradually increasing amount of load. The crutches are put forward in the normal way, and the injured leg moved forward to place the foot on the floor between them; pressing down to take most of the body-weight through the arms, the patient brings the other leg in front of the crutches. As the leg becomes stronger, more weight is taken through it and less on the arms. This allows the leg to become progressively more co-ordinated towards normal walking, without any risk of overload. The patient may progress to using one crutch or a walking stick, to maintain support for confidence, while taking most of the body-weight through the injured leg. The support has to be held on the opposite side to the injured leg, to avoid a limp which would put excessive pressure on the hip. Sometimes there is no need for this intermediate step of a single crutch or stick, and the patient returns to normal walking by abandoning the crutches.

Driving is out of the question, if it involves using the injured knee on pedal controls. The loss of normal co-ordination increases the risk of poor reactions in an emergency. In an accident, this could prejudice both the driver's innocence and full insurance cover. When the patient is being driven, the best position is reclining sideways on the back seat, with the injured leg fully supported on the seat. If the patient has to sit in the front of the car, both legs should be stretched out straight, with the foot of the uninjured leg ready to resist the pressure, in the event of sudden braking or an emergency stop. When the knee is recovering, the patient should try driving on traffic-free roads at first, if possible, in order to test how well the knee can perform sudden movements such as quick braking or gear changes. It is wise to regain confidence and driving skill, before going back to driving in normal traffic conditions.

9 Injuries to the Front of the Knee

TIBIAL TUBERCLE INJURIES

The tibial tubercle, the bump of bone just below the front of the knee at the top of the shin-bone, can be injured through overuse. The patellar tendon creates too much pressure at its attachment to the bone, causing gradually increasing pain. This happens through activities which involve repetitive loading of the knee through the quadriceps muscles, such as digging, squatting, running, especially on hills, hopping and jumping, squash and football. The problem may be triggered by an increase in the activity, for instance running further or more frequently, or playing football with a full-size ball instead of the child's smaller version. Heavy, muddy ground, or a particular camber can contribute, as can badly balanced shoes, or walking with a limp following a separate leg injury. The tibial tubercle can also be injured suddenly and traumatically. It may give way in a moment of overload, for instance when a weight-lifter tries to raise too heavy a weight from the deep-squat position, or it can be damaged by a direct blow over the bone, for instance in a fall onto the front of the knee, or if the bone is kicked, or hit by a hockey stick. A direct blow is extra painful if the tubercle has already been damaged by an overuse injury.

The damaged tibial tubercle is painful to touch or press. It also causes pain when the knee is bent under load, for instance when walking up or down stairs, or squatting. Kneeling can be very painful. Continuing the activity which has caused the pain, whether through overuse or trauma, makes the problem much worse.

Pain directly over the tibial tubercle usually involves some degree of disruption between the tubercle and the underlying shin-bone to which it is attached. In the child, this is a growth point, and the fusion process between the tubercle and the shin-bone takes place in the early teenage years. The tubercle is

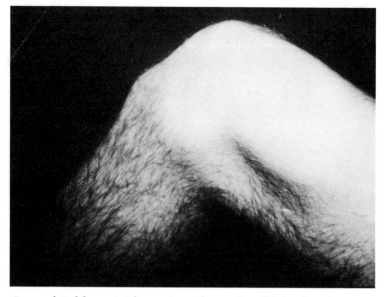

Osgood-Schlatter's 'disease' can leave the tibial tubercle abnormally prominent

especially vulnerable to overuse damage during this time, so the problem is particularly common in 12- to 16-year-olds, and it has a special name: Osgood-Schlatter's Disease. It is not a disease as such, but a mechanical problem. In the adult, the overuse mechanical disruption of the tibial tubercle is a type of stress fracture. It is similar in nature to the child's injury, except that the stress fracture problem is more easily cured, whereas the child's problem, if not properly managed, may develop into a weakened area which remains painful under stress well into adulthood. Apart from the tenderness, the tibial tubercle may look enlarged, and there may be noticeable fluid swelling around it. A severe tibial tubercle problem, whether it is a bad traumatic injury, or an overuse problem which has developed to a serious stage, can involve partial or total disruption of the tubercle, which is torn away, or avulsed, from its attachment on the shin-bone.

Having examined the painful knee, the doctor is likely to order X-rays to show whether the tubercle has been pulled away from its underlying bone. Bone scans may be done to show whether the bone is the cause of the pain, if the X-rays are normal. Once the diagnosis is established the doctor may recommend treatment from a physiotherapist, to maintain good muscles and function around the knee. If the tubercle has been badly disrupted, the doctor may refer to an orthopaedic surgeon, as it may be necessary to re-attach the tubercle to the shin-bone surgically.

If surgery is not needed, rest is the most important factor in curing tibial tubercle pain. For the child, this means restricting physical activities and sports to those which do not cause a painful reaction. The child's problem may take up to two years to cure itself completely, so few specialists recommend complete rest from sports, unless this is absolutely necessary. For the adult, rest from any painful activities for several weeks will usually allow the problem to clear up. Meanwhile, good muscle function around the knee must be maintained, so exercises which do not involve loading the knee are performed every day, such as those on pp. 24–27. Swimming and cycling can be useful ways of keeping fit while doing exercises which can help the knee. If inappropriate shoes have contributed to the problem, new shoes and protective insoles, possibly made up by a podiatrist, can help to relieve discomfort. Once the problem is cured, it is vital not to repeat the circumstances which brought on the injury, by avoiding overloading the knee, if possible, and by allowing for recovery days after any activities which have caused stiffness or fatigue to the knee or the quadriceps muscles.

PATELLAR TENDON INJURIES

Trauma can cause severe damage to the patellar tendon, tearing its fibres, sometimes right through. A complete tear is called a total rupture of the tendon. The injury involves a great stress, for instance a rough tackle and blocked kick in football, or a massive overload in lifting a heavy weight from the deep-squat position. It is an injury more likely to happen to sportsmen or manual workers who lift heavy loads. However, the tendon can give way under relatively minor stress if it has previously been weakened by overuse injuries or unwisely administered steriod injections.

When the patellar tendon tears, the victim feels an immediate pain and the tearing sensation. If the tear is right through the tendon, the knee-cap loses its anchor, and it may glide upwards on the thigh, creating a visible deformity to the knee.

80. Injuries to the Front of the Knee

At the moment of injury, ice can be applied to relieve pain and limit any swelling. If the pain is severe, the victim should have the knee bandaged from ankle to groin, and should be taken to hospital or to a doctor straight away. If the pain is not too acute, the knee should be bandaged, and the victim should see a doctor as soon as is convenient. If this involves some delay, ice should be re-applied at two- or four-hourly intervals, depending on the degree of swelling visible. If possible, painless movements should be performed, such as lying on the uninjured side and lifting the injured leg up sideways, or lying on the stomach, lifting the injured leg a little way backwards. If there is a complete tear, ice can be applied to reduce the pain, but the victim should immediately have the knee protected in a comfortable bandage and splint, and be carried to hospital. For the complete tear, it is most likely that the casualty surgeon or orthopaedic specialist would choose to re-attach the tendon immediately. For this reason, the victim should not be allowed to eat or drink anything between having the accident and seeing the doctors.

For the partial tear, or in the recovery phase following surgery to mend the completely torn tendon, the doctor is likely to refer the patient for physiotherapy, to improve the knee muscles and gradually regain full mobility through the quadriceps muscles and their tendon. Exercises would probably include some of those on pp. 35–38. Cycling and swimming are usually important elements in the rehabilitation programme, both for fitness and as valuable knee exercises.

Overuse injuries to the patellar tendon cause gradually increasing pain over the front of the knee. They are usually brought on by activities which involve loading the bent knee under the body's weight, as in hill running, hopping, jumping, lunging, kicking, squatting, digging, or moving up and down a ladder. As patellar tendon strain is particularly common among high- and long-jumpers, it is often called 'jumper's knee'. It could equally be termed 'squash player's knee', but it can be brought on by many sporting and everyday activities.

Any unusual or increased effort involving these activities can damage the patellar tendon, causing a tendonitis, or inflammation associated with an over-stretching or a degree of degeneration in the tendon. Sometimes, the tendon is not just strained but some of its fibres are partly torn. The bursa under the tendon (infrapatellar bursa) may become inflamed. Occasionally, one or both of the fat pads which lie on each side of the tendon become sore and painful as well. If the upper part of the tendon is involved, where it joins on to the tip of the knee-cap, the bone can be affected as well as the tendon: this is called Sinding-Larsen-Johansson's syndrome, after the two people who described it first. It is a type of osteochondritis, although its precise definition is still not properly understood by the experts. If the condition is allowed to develop to a severe stage, the tendon may tear off, or avulse, the tip of the knee-cap, either partly or completely. Another complication which can develop is calcification in the tendon, a deposit of hard tissue which can harden into a bone chip. Sometimes, the injured tendon tightens so much it pulls the knee-cap downwards, limiting its gliding movements and therefore stiffening the whole knee: this is called a patella baja.

In the early stages of overuse injury to the patellar tendon, the symptoms may be no more than a slight pain after the activity which is causing the problem. As the problem develops, pain is gradually felt during the activity as well as after it, although it may not be sufficient to make the activity impossible. However, the stage will gradually be reached when the tendon suffers from prolonged pain, and even normal movements such as walking become painful. The tendon then feels sore to press. If the tip of the knee-cap is involved, it feels extremely tender to the touch, and kneeling on it is very painful. The tendon tends to stiffen, and therefore can cause pain on being moved after being held still, for instance on rising after sitting down for a long period.

The doctor's examination includes tests to show whether the tendon hurts when it is under load, as in squatting movements, or straightening the knee with a resistance applied against the front of the ankle. If the tendon is stiffened, the full quadriceps stretch done lying on the stomach will be limited. If the problem is not severe, the doctor usually refers the patient for physiotherapy treatment, which will aim to reduce the pain and tenderness in the tendon, re-strengthen the knee's muscles, and regain full flexibility using exercises such as those on pp. 33–38. In more serious cases, for instance if X-rays show that there is calcification in the tendon, the doctor may refer the patient to an orthopaedic specialist, in case it eventually becomes necessary to free the tendon surgically. In all cases, rest from the pain-causing activity is an absolute priority in curing the problem, and a gradual, progressive return to normal is important in preventing a recurrence.

KNEE-CAP SYNDROMES

The joint between the knee-cap and the thigh-bone is a very common area of pain. The joint can become acutely painful because of a sudden traumatic injury, particularly if the knee-cap suffers a direct blow, such as a kick, a knock with a hockey stick, or a fall onto the bent knee. Gradual pain can come on in the knee-cap joint as a primary or secondary overuse condition. Primary overuse knee-cap pain is caused directly by activities which tend to load the bent knee, without allowing the knee muscles to balance the stresses sufficiently by straightening the knee. Kneeling, squatting, digging, balancing on a ladder, walking up and down long stairways or escalators, or even just sitting still for long periods can unbalance the knee muscles enough to cause knee-cap pain. The problem is very common among runners, especially those who do a lot of hill running, and joggers. It may be triggered by a particular run on a slope or camber. Sometimes the pain is caused or aggravated by poor foot mechanics, or inappropriate running shoes which throw the feet off balance. Knee-cap pain is often referred to as 'runner's knee', but it is also a common hazard of other sports, like downhill ski-ing, cycling with the saddle too low, rowing without straightening the knees fully at the end of the stroke, squash, and weight-training on knee extension machines without locking out the knees.

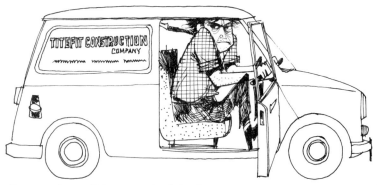

Cramped conditions are bad for knees

Primary knee-cap pain may appear in one or both knees. Sometimes it occurs first in one knee, and then affects the other later, because of overloading through compensation. Secondary knee-cap pain arises following other types of knee injury, such as cartilage tears, partly because the vastus medialis muscle which controls the inner side of the knee-cap is inhibited immediately in any traumatic injury to the knee, and needs careful retraining to regain its proper function, and partly because an injured knee is automatically held slightly bent for comfort, and this further weakens the muscles round the joint, especially vastus medialis. Occasionally the knee-cap is drawn and held downwards from its normal position, due to a complete tear in the muscles above the bone, or tightness in the patellar tendon below it. This condition is called a patella baja, and it can cause knee-cap pain because it limits the free gliding movements of the joint.

Pain from the knee-cap joint is felt over the front of the knee, either over the whole area, or over a particular point under, or close to, the knee-cap. When it first starts, the pain may only appear after the activity which is causing it, but as it develops, it becomes evident in many different situations when the knee is bent and bearing weight. Walking may cause pain, even on level surfaces, but the pain is worst going up or down stairs. Squatting and kneeling, especially for long periods, tend to cause pain. Sitting still for long periods may make the problem knee or knees ache: this is called the 'cinema sign'. Sometimes the pain is not felt while sitting, but on getting up from the seated position. The knee-cap may be tender if pressed. Grating and clicking sensations are typical features of knee-cap problems. Swelling does not necessarily appear, but if it does, it is usually just a puffiness around the knee-cap. Occasionally the knee-cap causes a sharp pain which makes the knee feel as though it is going to give way.

There are many pathologies, or particular types of damage, that can affect the back of the knee-cap or its receiving surface on the thigh-bone, and so give rise to knee-cap pain. Chondromalacia patellae is a common condition affecting the joint cartilage in the young, while older people may suffer from osteoarthritis, or degeneration in the knee-cap joint. The common factor underlying all the different types of knee-cap injury is pain arising from faulty movements in the joint, which allow the wrong parts of the joint surfaces to glide across each

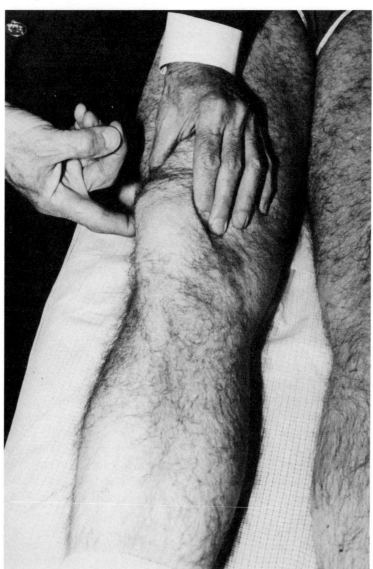

Feeling the undersurface of the knee-cap with the tip of the index finger

other, and which are caused by a mechanical imbalance in the muscles controlling the knee-cap's movements.

When the doctor examines the painful knee, or knees, the tests for vastus medialis efficiency (pp. 58–60) reveal the lack of

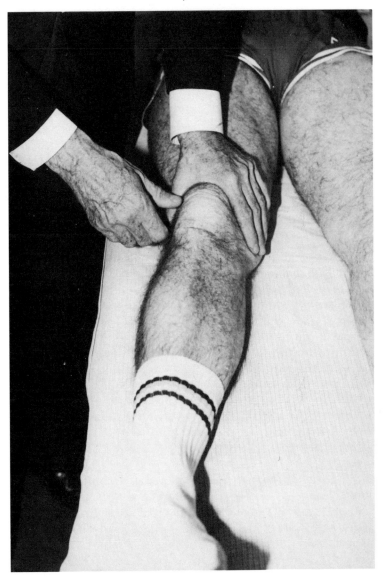

Clarke's sign

proper co-ordination between that muscle and the others around the knee. The knee-cap feels very tender when the doctor presses it down against the thigh-bone, while the patient sits, relaxed, on the couch, with legs straight. 'Clarke's sign' is another test performed with the patient sitting straight-legged on the couch: the doctor presses his hand against the top edge of the knee-cap, and blocks the movement, as the patient is asked to tighten the thigh muscles and twitch the knee-cap upwards. These tests are the main methods of confirming knee-cap syndrome by physical assessment. Further investigations may or may not be needed. X-rays may be taken to show possible damage to the bones in the knee-cap joint. The knee-caps may be X-rayed with the knees fully bent, to show not only the state of the bones, but also their position in relation to each other. Arthroscopy may be performed so that the surgeon can see the actual condition of the knee-cap joint, and any other damage in the rest of the knee complex.

Treatment of knee-cap pain is usually directed at the muscle imbalance which causes it. The knees should be actively straightened at frequent intervals during each day. For instance, people who sit down all day should try to stand up and lock their knees out at, perhaps, quarter- or half-hourly intervals. People who squat or kneel for long periods should stand up or sit with their legs straight whenever possible. Motorists should adjust the car seat so that their knees are as straight as possible when they depress the control pedals, and they should try to take frequent breaks to 'stretch their legs' on long journeys. Cyclists must make sure that their knees are almost straight as they push down on the pedals, by raising the saddle as high as is safe, and they should always stand up in the pedals when cycling uphill. Runners with knee-cap pain should avoid hills, cambers and slow jogging, until the problem is cured.

Supports for the knee can help knee-cap pain. The simplest support consists of a small piece of tubular bandage, almost four inches long, which is rolled over on itself into a band about half an inch wide, and then placed just below the tip of the knee-cap. This knee-cap strap helps to limit the full glide of the bone when the knee is bent and straightened. A more elaborate version of this strap, usually made of leather, can be bought. The most sophisticated type of support is a full knee brace, surrounding the knee, but open over the knee-cap, which aims to limit both the up-and-down glide and the sideways motion of the knee-cap.

Corrective exercises are essential to restoring the proper balance of muscles round the knee-cap. The recommended

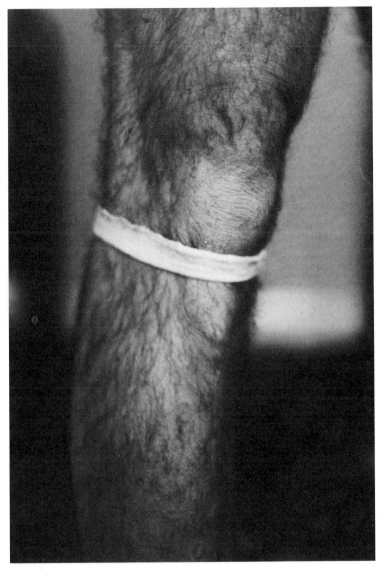

The knee-cap strap

exercise routine should be performed as frequently as possible, for instance between three and five times a day. The exercises should not cause pain, and should be built up gradually, for instance starting with five repetitions of each exercise, and building up in stages to five sets of ten. If the thigh muscles or the patellar tendon become sore through the corrective exercises, ice can be used to soothe the pain, and the quadriceps muscles should be stretched frequently (see exercises 3 and 4 on pp. 33–34), while the other corrective exercises should be cut back to just a few once or twice a day, but not abandoned. The exercises recommended to correct the muscle co-ordination usually include numbers 1 to 8 on pp. 24–26.

Knee-cap problems can usually be cured by conservative treatment, particularly physiotherapy, correcting the mechanical imbalance which causes the pain. If the mechanics can be corrected successfully, the problem knee stops causing pain, even though the particular damage in the joint may still be present. However, if a knee-cap problem is very severe or persistent, it may be necessary for the patient to be referred to an orthopaedic specialist with a view to surgery. Nowadays, it is relatively rare for the surgeon to scrape the back of the knee-cap, or remove the knee-cap completely, as used to be the standard procedures for chronic knee-cap problems. Recovery from this type of operation is a slow, arduous process. The more modern operations are aimed at correcting the mechanical imbalance round the knee-cap. One way of achieving this is to move the attachment point of the patellar tendon on the shin-bone; another is the lateral release operation, in which the covering of the muscles holding the outer side of the knee-cap is slit, in order to allow the knee-cap to shift towards the inner side of the knee, in better tracking alignment. Whichever type of corrective surgery is used, full recovery depends on rehabilitation exercises, preferably under the guidance of a physiotherapist.

KNEE-CAP DISLOCATION AND SUBLUXATION

When the knee-cap leaves its groove on the front of the thigh-bone, it is a sudden, traumatic injury. This injury usually occurs when the knee is bent and twisted with the body-weight over it, for instance in a sudden change of direction while running, or a fall down stairs. It is a particularly common problem in children and teenagers, especially if they are active in sports which involve a lot of running, bending and twisting, like field hockey, squash and football. If it happens when a child is very young, it tends to become a recurrent problem. The weak part of the knee-cap complex is almost always the

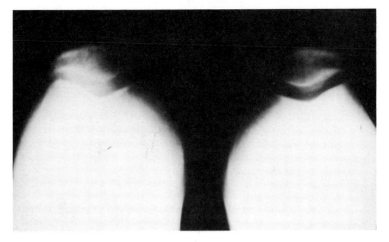

Subluxation: the knee-cap on the left of the picture is pulled outwards when the knee is fully bent

inner side, where the knee-cap is held in line mainly by the vastus medialis muscle. A movement which over-stresses the inner side of the knee can over-strain or tear the knee-cap's supporting structures, allowing the knee-cap to be pulled over to the opposite, outer side under the influence of the large outer quadriceps muscles. The injury happens more easily if the vastus medialis muscle has already been weakened, for instance due to inhibition associated with a previous knee injury or knee-cap pain. Occasionally, the problem is linked to the alignment of the thigh-bone on the shin-bone, especially in young girls with widely angled hips, and both knees may be prone to knee-cap dislocation. Growth spurts can be responsible for relative weakness in vastus medialis in boys and girls, and this can be another contributory factor to knee-cap dislocation.

At the moment when the knee-cap comes out of its groove, the victim is aware of something being 'out of place' in the knee. The pain is usually very sharp, and accompanied by a lot of swelling. If the knee-cap falls back into line immediately, the injury is called a subluxation. If it remains visibly out of place, it is a dislocation. The best course of action at the moment of injury is to use ice to relieve the pain and reduce the swelling, then bandage the knee comfortably, and transport the victim to hospital as quickly as possible. The doctor or surgeon will decide whether an operation is needed to restore stability. If surgery is not deemed necessary, it is likely that the knee will be protected in a plaster cast or full bandage for some weeks, and then treated with physiotherapy to regain full strength followed by mobility.

If medical help is not sought until the knee-cap has been injured several times, the general practitioner will probably refer the victim to an orthopaedic specialist. The diagnosis may not be quite clear at this late stage, so the specialist will probably check the knee for various possibilities. The victim may be aware that something goes out of place in the knee, but may also complain of pain over the front or inner side of the knee, and perhaps a feeling of 'giving way', which could indicate other knee conditions. One physical assessment test which indicates that the knee-cap tends to dislocate is the 'apprehension test', in which the victim sits over the end of the couch, with the specialist supporting the injured knee held straight; he then pushes the knee-cap gently towards the outer side of the knee, and gradually allows the knee to bend; at a certain angle, the knee-cap feels as though it is dislocating again, and the patient usually stops the specialist from bending the knee further.

If the problem has continued over a long period, each episode of dislocation tends to be more severe, and there comes a point where corrective surgery is inevitable. There are many different types of operation to give the knee-cap stability, so the choice remains with the surgeon, who generally explains to the patient what each procedure involves. Most of the operations aim to re-align the knee-cap and alter the angle between the knee-cap and the patellar tendon. After surgery, the priority in rehabilitation is to re-strengthen the knee muscles with special emphasis on vastus medialis (using exercises such as those on pp. 24–27). Mobility is then regained using exercises such as those on pp. 30–33. The final stage leading to full recovery, may include dynamic strengthening exercises (pp. 35–38) and then functional exercises (p. 38 or p. 39).

KNEE-CAP FRACTURES

Traumatic fracture, or a break, can happen if the knee-cap is subjected to severe direct violence, as in a fall from a height onto the bent knee, a car accident in which the knee hits the dashboard or steering wheel, a hard kick, or a heavy knock on the front of the knee from a hockey stick. The injury is extremely painful, and causes bruising and swelling, and possibly bleeding if the skin is broken. First-aid measures must be applied immediately, particularly to stem any bleeding with clean dressings. Cold compresses or ice bandages may be used to limit the swelling. The priority is to support the knee comfortably, perhaps by splinting the leg, holding the knee bent and supported on padding, and to have the victim transported to hospital immediately as a casualty. The casualty doctor or orthopaedic surgeon can then assess the extent of the damage through examination and X-rays, and decide whether the knee-cap needs immediate surgical repair, or whether it can heal simply through being protected in a plaster cast.

Stress fractures, or cracks which occur gradually through overuse, can happen to the knee-cap in young active people. Typically, pain is first noticed over the knee-cap after a particular activity which has involved repetitive movements, such as hopping and bounding exercises, hill running, or kicking practice for footballers. If the activity is continued, the pain gradually gets worse, although it disappears very quickly with rest, only to recur if normal sport is resumed too soon. The cause of the stress fracture is excessive muscle pull through the quadriceps muscle group against the knee-cap. Excessive, in this context, means an amount of stress for which the bone is unprepared, or not properly conditioned.

The symptoms may seem very similar to those of knee-cap pain, except that the knee-cap may feel very tender to the touch over its surface. The clue which helps the examining doctor to suspect a stress fracture is the background to the start of the pain, as, typically, the problem comes on with resumption of sport after a lay-off, or a sudden increase in training. In the early stages, confirming the stress fracture is difficult, because it does not necessarily show up on X-ray. Therefore, if the doctor suspects a stress fracture, he is most likely to recommend rest from any painful activities for several weeks, to allow the bone to recover, coupled with continued exercises of any kind which do not cause pain, such as conditioning training, swimming and cycling. When the pain and tenderness have subsided completely, a gradual return to sport is allowed, with special care to avoid doing the same type of repetitive training on consecutive days. Allowing rest days for recovery from repetitive stress, during which different types of activity can be performed, is a key factor in avoiding a recurrence of the stress fracture.

The knee-cap stress fracture can develop to a serious stage in which the bone is actually pulled apart, so that a visible break appears on X-rays. This happens if the sufferer ignores the initial warning symptoms of gradually increasing pain over the bone, associated with a particular sport. When the bone breaks, the injury is sudden and traumatic, and the casualty should be taken to hospital as quickly as possible. The casualty doctor or orthopaedic surgeon can then decide whether surgical repair is needed. The injury is very similar to the traumatic fracture, except that it happens without particular violence to the knee, and it may even, at first sight, appear to happen without any warning.

Although the cause of the stress fracture is always an increase in a repetitive physical activity, various factors can influence or aggravate the injury, such as foot or knee mechanics, and previous injuries which have affected the efficiency of the knee muscles. The knee-cap itself may be affected by a congenital condition called the bipartite or tripartite patella, in which the knee-cap's separate parts fail to grow together properly in childhood, and remain distinct. The fact that the knee-cap consists of parts or has a separate fragment in its structure may never cause any problems, but in the context of a repetitive sporting activity, it may make the knee-cap more vulnerable to stress fractures or traumatic fractures which develop from stress fractures.

'HOUSEMAID'S KNEE' (PREPATELLAR BURSITIS)

The fluid-filled pouch, or bursa, which lies over the lower part of the knee-cap, separating it from the skin, can be inflamed traumatically through a direct blow. This could be a kick in football, a hit from a hockey stick, a blow as the knee hits the dashboard in a car accident, or a fall onto the bent knee. The bursa can also become inflamed more gradually, as a type of overuse injury. This can be the result of excessive direct pressure or friction over the front of the knee. The condition was called 'housemaid's knee' because it was an occupational hazard for women who knelt down and moved around on their knees to scrub floors. Other people who kneel a great deal in

HOUSEMAID'S KNEE

their work, such as carpet-layers and electricians, have a similar risk of irritating the bursa.

When the bursa is inflamed, it forms an egg-like swelling over the front of the knee. In the initial stage of a traumatic bursitis, the swelling may feel hot and look red. In the later stages, or if the swelling has been appearing at intervals through overuse, the bursa may not feel very painful. It may just restrict the full bending movement of the knee, by pulling on the skin when squatting movements are performed, or the quadriceps muscles are fully stretched.

If the bursitis interferes with normal activities, it should be examined by the victim's doctor. As the bursitis can occur spontaneously, as part of an inflammatory condition, the doctor would wish to establish its cause first of all. If the problem is purely a mechanical one, the treatment for it depends on how badly the bursitis affects the patient. If there is not too much pain or movement restriction, it may be sufficient to protect the knee from further friction by avoiding kneeling on it and avoiding direct pressure. Applying ice once or twice a day, and wearing a comfortable padded bandage may help to limit the swelling, and possibly even to reduce it. The knee's muscles must be maintained, especially through isometric exercises, and it should be kept as mobile as possible, without causing pain and further inflammation by forcing the bending movement. For more severe cases, the doctor may decide to drain the fluid out of the bursa, or to refer the patient to an orthopaedic specialist, with a view to having the inflamed bursa cut out surgically. The bursa may recur after drainage or removal, making further treatment necessary, if the recurrence is bad enough. In all cases, the doctor may decide to refer the patient for physiotherapy treatment to help maintain or improve the knee function.

QUADRICEPS MUSCLE INJURIES

The quadriceps muscles can be injured close to the front of the knee, either on or just above their attachment to the top of the knee-cap. A traumatic injury can cause a strain, tear or bruise in the muscles. Damage can be caused by a sudden over-contraction, for instance in a fall while walking down stairs, running forwards or jumping upwards, or in a blocked tackle in football. The lower thigh can suffer a direct blow in a variety of different sports or everyday activities, and this can cause a deep bruising in the quadriceps muscles, with additional tearing of the muscle fibres if the muscles were contracting when they were hit. If the leg is hit by a sharp implement, like an ice-skate or the edge of a ski, the muscles may be cut through. Overuse injuries can cause gradually increasing pain in the quadriceps muscles, associated with repetitive activities, for instance walking, crouching, running, breast-stroke swimming, training for jumping events, or kicking practice for football. Overuse strains may be influenced or triggered by muscle fatigue, cold, cramp, and previous injuries affecting the mechanics of the leg joints or the overall co-ordination of the leg's muscle groups.

In a traumatic injury there is immediate pain and perhaps bleeding, possibly followed by some bruising and swelling over the injured area, depending on the type and severity of the injury. First-aid consists of applying clean dressings to stop any bleeding. Ice packs or cold compresses are used to reduce the pain and limit any swelling or internal bruising. If there is a lot of swelling, a soft, compressive bandage over the whole area helps to keep the leg comfortable and control the effusion. On no account should the muscles be rubbed or massaged in the immediate or early stages of the injury, as there is a danger that this would cause a condition called myositis ossificans in the muscle, in which bone pieces form within the muscle fibres. If the injury is severe, the victim should be taken to hospital immediately. If the muscle has been cut through or completely ruptured, for instance, it may be necessary to stitch it together surgically. The examining doctor checks whether there is a visible gap in the muscle bulk, and whether the patient is capable of lifting the leg straight up at all. A badly torn or strained muscle may be accompanied by bone injury, so the doctor may check for fractures through X-rays. A complete tear of the attachment of the muscles to the upper part of the knee-cap can cause the condition called 'patella baja', in which the knee-cap is bound down below its normal position. If surgical repair has been necessary, the surgeon dictates the phases of recovery. In many cases, with or without surgery, early movement is considered essential for a good recovery, so the patient is encouraged to perform as much knee-bending and straightening motion as is comfortable, usually under the guidance of a physiotherapist. Sometimes a machine is used to provide continuous movement for the knee while the patient is still in bed after the operation. As flexibility returns, the muscles are gradually re-strengthened, using exercises with increasing weight-resistance and range of movement.

The overuse injury to the quadriceps muscles usually has few external signs, such as bruising or swelling, although the muscles may be tender to touch. The doctor should be told how the pain first started and how it has developed. The muscle strain is usually confirmed by testing the resisted movements of the quadriceps, which show pain as the patient straightens the knee while the doctor blocks the movement with his hand. The muscles also feel tight, compared to the uninjured side, when the quadriceps are put on full stretch: squatting down may cause pain, or the tightness may be revealed when the patient lies prone and the doctor pushes the patient's heel gently towards the buttocks. Once the overuse injury is confirmed, he is likely to refer the patient for physiotherapy, which would aim to restore flexibility to the muscles, then power and co-ordination, before a gradual return to normal physical activities can be allowed. The exercise programme includes stretching (p. 33, exs 3 and 4) and mobilising (pp. 30–32. exs 1–10), followed by strengthening work (pp. 35–38), and finally functional exercises such as those on pp. 38 or 39.

10 Internal Injuries to the Knee

CARTILAGE INJURIES

The knee's soft buffering cartilages (menisci) can be injured traumatically by jarring or twisting stresses. Abnormal pressure may occur when the knee is bent and twisted, or when it is straight and forced backwards or sideways. One, or even both of the cartilages may split or tear, through being trapped between the thigh- and shin-bones. This type of traumatic injury can happen, for instance, in a fall down stairs; to the footballer in a tackle; to the downhill skier who falls awkwardly; to the squash player who turns too sharply; to the gardener who over-balances while crouching; or to the truck driver who lands straight-legged when he jumps down from his cab. Traumatic injury to the cartilages usually involves a recognisable or awkward movement, which cannot be foreseen or avoided. However, some activities make the cartilages particularly vulnerable to traumatic injury, by placing special stress on them, so that only slight extra stress is needed to cause damage. Examples of this include full squatting movements under heavy load in weightlifting, or the 'frog-sitting' stretching exercise often used by breast-stroke swimmers, in which the knees are held twisted through kneeling, sitting back on the haunches, with the feet tucked on either side of the hips, rather than straight under the seat.

The cartilages are more easily injured in older people, because the cartilage plates, or bone coverings within the knee joint, become thinner with age, and therefore lose their ability to absorb shock efficiently. Sports players may make themselves more vulnerable to cartilage injuries by failing to warm up properly, because the bony cartilage plates temporarily thin down when a person has been sitting still for some time, and they only restore themselves to their full shock-absorbing function after the knee has been exercised. If the knee is put under excessive or abnormal stress before the cartilage plates have been re-vitalised by warm-up exercises, the soft-tissue cartilages may be overloaded. Congenital defects can make the cartilages specially vulnerable to injury. For instance, some people are born with cartilages which are almost completely round and solid, rather than crescent-shaped: these are called discoid cartilages, and the extra thickness in the centre of the cartilage is easily damaged through pressure from the knee's bone ends, especially in active children. Sometimes an extra fold of synovial lining tissue, called a plica, can cause symptoms very similar to those of a torn cartilage, by 'catching' in the joint on certain movements. The plica is normally identified and treated in the same way as the damaged cartilage.

The cartilages may also suffer overuse damage, causing gradual pain. Wear-and-tear degeneration in older people may be the result of the cumulative loading the cartilages have suffered over the years. Younger people may have cartilage degeneration problems if their knees have been subjected to very heavy loading, as in heavy weightlifting, long-distance running, or heavy manual labouring, especially if they started performing these activities during the vulnerable growth phases of their teenage years. Overuse damage may be the long-term result of previous, minor injuries to the cartilages. It may also occur if the normal mechanics of the knee have been altered, either by injuries or by postural habits affecting the normal muscle balance round the joint. Occasionally, cysts form on the cartilage, which may cause no problems, unless they become big enough to interfere with the knee's function. If damaged parts of the cartilage break off, they may form loose bodies in the knee, which intermittently block the joint's movements.

Cartilage pain may be severe at first, if it is caused by a bad injury, but it may recede to an ache if it has lasted for some time, or if the damage is of the overuse type. The pain is usually perceived as being 'inside the knee', although it may seem to be more to the front, back or sides of the joint. Sometimes the pain only occurs when the knee is in a certain position. Knee swelling is usually evident in cartilage injuries: it may vary from a tiny pocket of fluid over one point of the knee, to a gross swelling all round the joint. Often, in a traumatic injury, the swelling only appears some hours after the accident. If there is a cyst on the cartilage, it may protrude to form a visible lump on the surface of the knee. Cartilage damage may make the knee feel weak or unstable, but more often it causes clicking in the joint, or a total locking in which the knee gets stuck in a certain position, and can only be freed by a manipulation, usually a twisting movement.

First-aid in the traumatic cartilage injury consists of ice applications to reduce the pain and swelling. The whole leg should be comfortably bandaged, preferably with the knee straight, and the victim should be transported to hospital. If at all possible, the victim should try to do some static exercises for the thigh muscles virtually straight away, even if this involves simply twitching the knee-cap (p. 24). The doctor or surgeon who examines the knee wants to know exactly what happened, and which way the knee moved in the accident. Immediately after a traumatic injury, the knee may be too painful and swollen to test. The orthopaedic surgeon may decide to do an arthroscopy immediately, for a certain diagnosis, and with a view to operating on the cartilage if necessary, or he may wait to let the symptoms settle, in order to assess the knee at a later stage. If the knee is badly swollen, he may drain off, or aspirate, the fluid. The knee is protected from further damage by a full-length bandage or plaster cast which holds the leg straight. The patient has to start doing static exercises (pp. 24–27) straight away, and maintain a daily routine of them until the knee is ready for further rehabilitation.

Once the initial soreness has abated, or if he is seeing the injured knee at a late stage, the surgeon performs the tests which may indicate whether a cartilage is torn. He may go on to have X-rays and arthrograms taken, to identify any bone, cartilage or other soft tissue damage. Arthroscopy may be performed, possibly to confirm the diagnosis, or with a view to operating on the injured cartilage. Occasionally, the surgeon chooses to use a slightly different testing method to confirm cartilage damage in a knee which has been injured for a long time: he may refer the patient to a physiotherapist for so-called 'provocative exercises' which are designed to stress the knee in order to show up locking or movement limitations in the joint.

Once a cartilage is torn, it will not mend itself. At best, the broken part of the cartilage does not interfere with the knee's normal function. Otherwise, the injured cartilage causes continuing episodes of pain and swelling, and often of locking. If the knee is symptom-free, the patient may be given physiotherapy treatment to make the muscle protection as good as

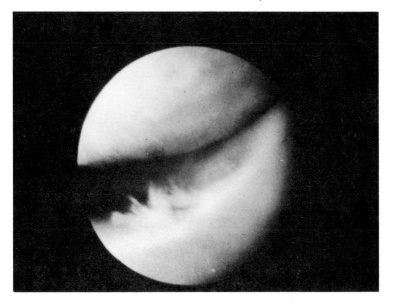

A torn cartilage, seen through the arthroscope

possible, before returning to normal activities. If the cartilage causes functional problems, there is little option but to have the damaged part removed surgically. The cartilage removal operation is called a meniscectomy. Nowadays, if the surgeon decides to operate to remove the torn cartilage, he normally tries to do so through the arthroscope, as recovery is so quick. It is possible for the patient to be discharged from hospital on the same day as the operation, although it is more common to wait for a day or two, by which time walking is fairly comfortable. Normal activities can often be resumed within a fortnight, although it is not advisable for sportsmen to return to demanding contact sports like football or rugby without a slightly longer period of rehabilitation. If it is not possible to remove the damaged part of the cartilage efficiently through the arthroscope, the surgeon uses the traditional method of opening up the knee with a scar (arthrotomy). The knee has to be held stiff for ten to fourteen days after this operation, to allow the scar to heal, so recovery is slower than after the arthroscopy. Full recovery may take up to three months or occasionally even longer.

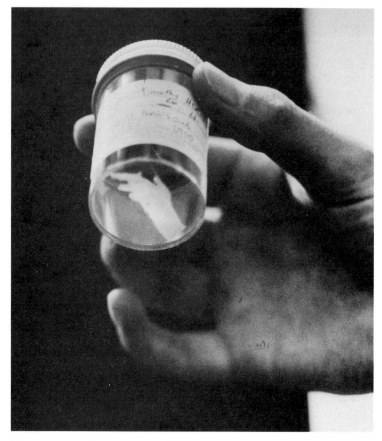

The torn cartilage removed

Rehabilitation exercises are begun immediately after the cartilage injury, and immediately after any corrective surgery. In the first phase of recovery, the static exercises (pp. 24–27) are used. After arthroscopy, the knee is mobilised within the first few days, despite the swelling that inevitably remains in the joint from the operation. If the knee has been opened up, knee bending exercises are normally avoided if any swelling persists, so they may be deferred until some three or four weeks after the operation. The third recovery phase consists of knee strengthening exercises involving joint movement (pp. 35–38), and the final phase leads into full recovery for normal everyday activities (p. 38), or, for the sportsman, fitness work simulating the demands of the individual's sport (p. 39).

Progress through the four recovery phases is dictated by the absence of painful reactions to the graded exercises. If the knee is allowed to recover its full strength and mobility, the risk of re-injury or a secondary related injury is reduced. When a damaged cartilage is removed surgically, the knee loses part of its buffering shock-absorbers. In fact, the cartilage normally grows back again within about two years, and its absence is not detrimental to good knee function. But it is unwise to over-stress the knee too soon after cartilage surgery, even though arthroscopy makes recovery seem deceptively quick and easy. The knee can only be considered safe when it has recovered full co-ordination, and time must be allowed for this.

CRUCIATE LIGAMENT INJURIES

The cruciate ligaments in the centre of the knee can only be injured by a strong shearing force across the knee, which may be a twisting stress, sideways pressure, or a jarring force which makes the knee bend backwards. This is a traumatic injury which can happen in everyday life, for instance in a fall down stairs or stepping down from a height, but it is a particular risk in contact field sports like soccer, rugby, or hockey.

It is possible to tear through both the cruciate ligaments, but it is more common for only one to be injured. Other structures are often injured with the cruciate ligament, such as one or both cartilages (menisci), or the knee's outer ligaments. The degree of damage to the cruciate ligament can vary from a slight over-stretch which loosens the ligament, in a relatively minor injury, to a complete tear which cuts through the centre of the ligament, or detaches one of the ends from its attachment onto the top of the shin-bone or the bottom of the thigh-bone. The injury is always painful, and sometimes the victim hears or feels a 'snap' as the ligament tears. Swelling is usually evident after the injury.

As this is a serious knee injury, the diagnosis has to be established as quickly as possible after the injury. The casualty surgeon or orthopaedic surgeon who sees the victim as an emergency may decide to perform an arthroscopy immediately, to find out the extent of the damage. If the cruciate ligament is torn, the surgeon may decide to repair it immediately, if this is feasible and likely to restore good stability to the knee. If the ligament is not badly damaged, or if the

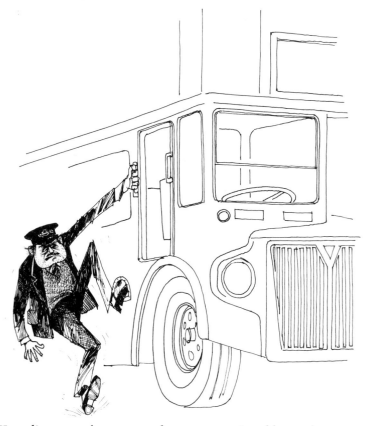

Knee ligament damage can be an occupational hazard

repair is not likely to be successful, the surgeon may opt to protect the knee in a cast, and put the patient through a full rehabilitation programme. If this fails to restore stability in the long-term, the surgeon will review the situation, and decide then whether any of the various possible operations will make good the damage.

If the diagnosis is not established immediately, and remedial exercises are not followed avidly, the knee will continue to give rise to symptoms several months after the injury. When the cruciate ligament is damaged or torn, and functional stability is not regained, either through surgical repair or through muscle strengthening, the knee feels unstable, and tends to give way when it is held at certain angles with the body's weight over it.

It may give, for instance, when the victim walks down stairs, if the foot is turned in a particular way; or it may be sufficient for the victim to turn slightly awkwardly while standing upright. The direction of the instability depends on which of the cruciate ligaments is damaged, and which part of the ligament. The degree of instability depends on the severity of the damage. Every time the knee gives way or causes a sharp stab of pain, it tends to swell up perceptibly.

If the knee is assessed at a late stage following the injury, the orthopaedic specialist usually goes through the physical tests for the knee's stability, especially the rotatory tests, including the 'pivot shift' (p. 61). X-rays and arthrograms may be ordered, or the surgeon may decide to establish the diagnosis by performing an arthroscopy. If the diagnosis of cruciate damage is confirmed, the surgeon has to decide whether to repair the ligament surgically, or whether to rely on a protective rehabilitation programme. There are many different types of operation for damaged cruciate ligaments, involving direct stitching or re-attachment of the ligament, replacement by other tissues or artificial fibres, or tightening other structures round the knee to compensate for the loss of the cruciate's function. Very often, the surgeon cannot guarantee that a particular operation will be totally successful. This is why a full

Anterior drawer test

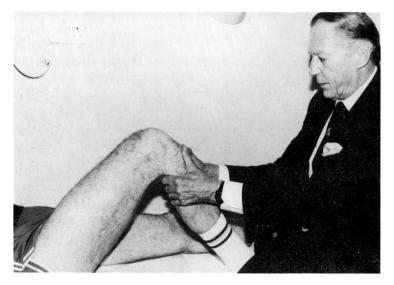

months in the initial phase. If the functional recovery is not complete, the brace may become a permanent feature in the victim's active life, if he or she wishes to continue demanding sports like ski-ing. The mobile brace, made-to-measure for the victim, may support the knee sufficiently to safeguard the joint and make it painfree in relatively dangerous situations.

KNEE BONE FRACTURES

The shin-bone and the thigh-bone are extremely strong, but they can be broken by a violent force. When they break close to the knee joint, the joint's soft-tissue structures, such as the capsule and ligaments, are often damaged at the same time. This type of serious traumatic injury can happen through a direct blow, for instance an awkward fall from a height such as a ladder; through a crush injury, for instance if a car runs over the leg, or when a horse falls sideways, trapping the rider's leg; or through shearing stress, for instance when a skier has a bad twisting fall, and the boot bindings fail to release, trapping the foot.

Fractures can be described in various categories. A simple fracture is a broken bone without a skin wound. An open fracture involves a skin wound, while a compound fracture is one in which the broken bone is visible through the skin wound. A comminuted fracture means that the bone has shattered, rather than having a single break line. An impacted, or compressed fracture means that the broken bone has been crushed on itself. In an avulsion fracture, a bone fragment is torn away when a tendon or ligament holds under stress, but breaks off its attachment point on the bone. If the joint cartilage (bone covering) is damaged with the bone, it is an osteochondral fracture. Greenstick fractures happen to children, when the damaged bone cracks and bends rather than breaking right through, because of its natural resilience. A complicated fracture involves damage to other structures besides the bone, such as blood vessels or nerves.

If the knee bones, separately or together, are obviously or probably fractured, the first-aid priority is to stop any bleeding. Both bones contain marrow, which forms and stores blood, so a break causes a heavy loss of blood. Any wounds should be covered with clean dressings, to try to minimise the risk of infection in or near the broken bone. The leg should then be immobilised and protected in a splint, so that the casualty can be transported to hospital. The casualty or orthopaedic surgeon then analyses the damage, and decides the best method of aligning the bones into the best position for functional healing. A plaster cast may be sufficient protection, or the bones may need stabilising with plates or screws, or bedrest with the leg fixed in traction may be used. A broken bone starts to heal immediately after the accident, but it takes up to three months for a leg bone to heal and become partly usable, and a further three months for re-strengthening. Full recovery usually takes up to a year. The process can be even longer, if complications such as infections delay the healing process. If plates or screws are used to make the bone stable initially, it may become necessary to remove them, in a further operation at a later stage, if they cause any discomfort.

From the beginning of the recovery process, protective exercises are performed at very frequent intervals throughout the day, usually under the guidance of a physiotherapist. Recovering the use of the leg is most efficiently done through progressive remedial exercises, so that, for instance, the muscles are as strong as possible before the leg is used for walking again. Fractures close to the knee-joint inevitably affect the joint itself, causing stiffness and weakness, and rehabilitation has to be directed towards correcting knee function, as well as helping the leg as a whole to work. In the first stage of active recovery, when the patient is allowed out of bed, the leg is generally protected from taking weight, so the patient uses crutches. Gradually, the foot is put to the ground, although weight-bearing is minimised by the crutches. The leg gradually regains strength through exercises and increasing weight-bearing, so that the patient progressively returns to normal. If the person's normal activities involve heavy manual work, or elements of danger, as in roofing or climbing electricity pylons, or contact sports such as football or karate, the final recovery phase has to be approached cautiously. There is always a risk of re-fracturing the leg, if it is overloaded suddenly before it is completely ready.

Stress fractures are bone cracks caused as an overuse injury. This type of fracture always happens as the result of a repetitive activity, which overloads the affected bone through excessive, attritional muscle pull. One's bones are only as strong as they need to be. They may be weakened through lack of use, for instance by a long period in bed for illness, through hormonal changes such as the menopause, or through old age. Even an unusually long walk may be enough to cause a stress fracture in a vulnerable person. The problem is common to sports which involve repetitive training, such as marathon running. Any change in the amount of repetitive movement involved in the sport can cause a stress fracture, such as intensive training after a lay-off, or increased training building up to a race. This type of fracture can happen anywhere on any bone, and its precise location depends on which muscles have exerted the excess pressure, and the angle at which these muscles pull against the affected bone.

Round the knee, stress fractures can happen in the front, back or sides of the shin-bone or thigh-bone, and they can affect the top, or head, of the fibula at the side of the knee. The victim feels a gradually increasing pain in the affected bone, related directly to the repetitive activity which causes the problem. The pain may come on immediately after the activity at first, and may be noticeable at night, but as it gets worse it becomes more evident during the repetitive activity. Characteristically, the pain disappears completely with a few days' rest, but it recurs quickly if long walks or running training are resumed.

The doctor who examines the leg must be given an accurate picture of how the pain came on, as this is essential to identifying the stress fracture, and differentiating it from the other possible causes of similar pain. X-rays, in the early stages, do not show up the damage in this kind of stress fracture, whereas a bone scan does. An X-ray usually only confirms the stress fracture once the bone is healing, and healing can only take place when the bone has had several weeks of rest from the pain-causing activity, although any exercise which does not cause pain should be continued. The runner, for instance, may find that court games like squash or badminton do not hurt the injured leg, because of the variety of leg movements involved. It is rare for the specialist to immobilise the stress fracture in a plaster cast, as total protection can further weaken the bone, and prevent healing. Provided any painful activities are avoided for up to twelve weeks, or until a check bone scan shows that healing has taken place, the stress fracture will heal. If the victim tries to ignore the pain and continue normal running training, for instance, there is a risk that eventually the bone will break completely. Once the bone has healed, it is important to avoid the situation that caused the problem, by building up to any repetitive physical activities like walking or running in a gradual process. Marathon runners, for instance, should allow recovery days between running sessions, and should use alternative training, such as weight-training, conditioning workouts, swimming, cycling or other sports to keep fit and to counterbalance the repetitive stresses involved in running.

Epiphyseal fractures are a particular complication of broken bones in children and teenagers. The top of the shin-bone and the lower end of the thigh-bone are both growth points in the young. If they are badly disrupted in an accident which breaks or cracks the bones, or if they suffer overuse damage associated with stress fractures, there may be a long-term effect on the bone growth. Osteochondritis dissecans is another complication of bone injury in young people: if the joint cartilage is damaged, perhaps by repeated minor trauma or through a shearing injury which pulls away the cruciate ligament attachment, the cartilage can break up to form fragments, or loose bodies, in the knee. The doctor normally refers this type of problem to an orthopaedic specialist for detailed advice and management.

KNEE JOINT DISLOCATION

The main knee joint can be pulled out of line by a severe traumatic injury which breaks through the joint's binding ligaments and capsule covering. The dislocation means that the shin-bone and thigh-bone ends no longer face each other. As it is always a serious accident, dislocation is often accompanied by bone fracture in either or both of the bones. Dislocation can happen in any of the knee's directions of movement, so the shin-bone can be pulled forwards or backwards relative to the thigh-bone, if the cruciate ligaments or joint capsule tear; if the inner (medial) and outer (lateral) ligaments give way, the dislocation may be sideways; if most of the knee bindings tear at the same time, the shin and thigh-bones may be twisted out of place.

This type of injury can only happen if the knee is subjected to a very violent force, as can happen in football, if a player falls across an opponent's outstretched leg, or if a rider is pinned down in a fall while the horse rolls over the rider's knee. The injury is usually extremely painful immediately, but occasionally there is relatively little pain, and the victim only realizes the knee has been injured when it stiffens and becomes painful later on. At the moment of injury, the best treatment is immediate replacement of the joint into its proper line, if a qualified doctor happens to be present. On no account should the knee be manipulated by an unqualified person, as this can cause serious damage. Safe first-aid consists of applying ice to reduce the pain, supporting the knee comfortably, and having the victim transported immediately to hospital.

Even if the dislocation has gone back into place immediately, the victim should still be sent to hospital as an emergency. A major displacement of the knee bones can cause serious damage to the main arteries which lie close to the joint, especially the popliteal artery which runs vertically down the back of the knee. The casualty doctor needs to examine the injured joint as quickly as possible, to find out if the blood vessels are damaged, so that surgical repair can be done immediately, if necessary. Otherwise, there is a risk, in the unluckiest of cases, that the leg could develop gangrene and have to be amputated. Another secondary complication which can arise in knee joint dislocations, especially if the bones are pressed sideways or twisted, is damage to the nerve which lies close to the outer side of the knee, the lateral popliteal branch of the common peroneal nerve. This can cause a paralysis of some of the leg muscles, leading to an inability to lift the foot upwards, a condition called 'foot-drop'. The surgeon would operate to try to repair the nerve, at the same time as manipulating the joint back into place, and trying to mend the torn ligaments and joint capsule.

Recovery from knee joint dislocation often involves having the knee protected in a cast for several months, while muscle strength is gradually rebuilt, usually under the guidance of a physiotherapist. Particular care has to be taken to protect the circulation, so the leg has to be rested with the foot up and supported on a soft cushion, whenever possible. If there is any sign of constriction in the cast, or burning discomfort, a doctor must be seen immediately. Once the surgeon allows the cast to be removed, mobility is gradually increased, although the knee is unlikely to regain its full bending movement. However, recovery can still be good enough to allow most normal activities.

OSTEOARTHRITIS AND DEGENERATIVE ARTHRITIS

Osteoarthritis is a condition in which joint surfaces suffer inflammation and subsequently degenerate. A person can suffer from widespread osteoarthritis affecting several of the body's joints, including the small joints of the fingers and thumbs, the spinal joints, the shoulders, the hips and the knees. It is not simply the result of wear and tear: it can be a hereditary condition. Various factors can contribute to the onset of osteoarthritis, including obesity; varicose veins; poor joint mechanics (such as a limp, or pigeon-toed gait, which can distort the function of the hips and knees); a prolonged period of total immobility, for instance if a joint is protected in plaster and the patient placed on bed-rest because of joint disease or infection; or excessive muscle development (such as a weight-lifter's enlarged thighs, which place abnormal compressive forces on the knees). A degree of osteoarthritis, or joint degeneration, is said to affect one or more joints in the majority of people over 60, but people who have inherited a predisposition to osteoarthritis may suffer at a much younger age. For the sake of specific definitions, specialists often call the type of deterioration due to mechanical causes such as injuries 'degenerative arthritis', and reserve the term 'osteoarthritis' for the inherited, progressive disease process, although the joint changes are the same.

Joint inflammation followed by degeneration can be the delayed result of previous injury or infection. Degeneration in the knee joint may follow an injury which happened several years previously. It is more likely to follow injury if there was blood in the joint at the time of the trauma, and it was not removed (aspirated) quickly; if the injury altered the joint's normal mechanics; if it caused repeated episodes of locking or giving way; if it was not diagnosed properly and quickly; or if recovery from the injury was not complete. Degenerative change in the knee is also common following the cartilage removal operation (meniscectomy), probably because of the alteration in joint mechanics following this procedure.

The inflammation of osteoarthritis affects the articular cartilage (bone covering) in a joint first, but if it develops, the bone at the edges of the cartilage or underlying it can be involved. In the knee, as in other joints, the joint may become narrower than normal because of the degeneration; the rounded edge of the thigh-bone knuckle (condyle) may become flattened and enlarged; jutting points of bone, called osteophytes, may form in the joint; or a ridge of bone may form at the edge of the affected area in the joint. These degenerative changes show up on X-ray, and confirm the presence of osteoarthritis. Sometimes parts of the joint surface crack and break off, forming small cavities (erosions) and loose bodies in the joint. In the main knee joint, these changes may happen on either side, affecting the inner (medial) or outer (lateral) parts of the joint separately, or both together.

Osteoarthritis and degenerative arthritis do not necessarily cause pain. Sometimes a joint can look very severely damaged through osteoarthritic changes on X-ray, but it is completely painless in normal activities. The osteoarthritic knee usually stiffens progressively, losing the ability to bend or straighten fully. It may look deformed: in a mild case the knee may be held just slightly bent, with the shin-bone a little twisted; severe osteoarthritis may make the leg bow outwards or inwards, with a more noticeable degree of twisting through the shin-bone. The direction of the deformity depends on the area

A loose body, seen through the arthroscope

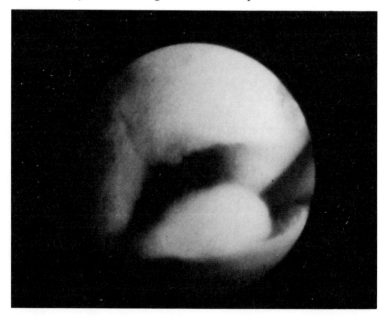

of damage. If the inner (medial) part of the knee is affected, the knee tends to bow outwards (genu varum), while the shin-bone may twist inwards. Osteoarthritis in the outer (lateral) part of the joint tends to bow the knee inwards into the knock-knee position (genu valgum), with some outward twisting of the shin-bone. When the whole knee joint is affected, the knee tends to become progressively more bent, in a position called a fixed flexion deformity. There may also be some bowing, if one side of the knee is worse than the other. When the knee joint space has become very narrow, the knee feels lax, because its ligaments do not shorten to take up the slack.

If osteoarthritis does cause discomfort as well as movement limitation, it varies from an ache to persistent severe pain. Sometimes, a minor injury triggers pain in the knee, showing up osteoarthritis which has been present in the joint for some time. Otherwise, osteoarthritic pain tends to build up gradually. The pain is usually worst in weight-bearing activities, such as walking, kneeling, running or jumping, but it may be present at night, and the knee or knees may also ache during sitting. Wet or cold weather may increase the pain, but the affected joint may also be aggravated by heat, whether through hot weather, too many bedclothes, or the application of heat rubs.

Protecting the knee from overload and poor mechanics is important in limiting or preventing the pain of osteoarthritis. The overweight victim must reduce through a properly balanced diet coupled with moderate exercise, preferably under the guidance of a dietician and a physiotherapist. Movement is important for the osteoarthritic knee: sitting still all day can make the pain very much worse by increasing the joint stiffness. Flexibility needs to be maintained through gentle mobilizing exercises and stretching for all the muscle groups of the thigh (pp. 30–35). Strength should be maintained and improved in the muscles, using both the isometric exercises holding the knee straight (pp. 24–27), and the weight-resisted exercises involving some knee movement (pp. 35–38). The sedentary person should try to stretch the legs at frequent intervals, possibly every ten minutes during the day: this can mean simply straightening the knee to lift the foot off the floor, then gently lowering it several times; straightening the knee with the heel on the floor to lock the knee out; or standing up and walking around. The labourer doing heavy work may have to take up lighter duties, or even change jobs. Taking up exercise like swimming, cycling or Yoga stretching can be beneficial. Jarring through the leg has to be prevented, as much as possible. Shock-absorbing polymer insoles provide protection during walking or running. If faulty foot mechanics have contributed to poor knee movements, specially fitted corrective insoles from a podiatrist can help.

For the sportsman, normal sport can be continued, provided it does not cause or aggravate the pain, either during exercise sessions or afterwards. Sports involving a lot of jarring or compression on the affected knee may have to be limited. For instance the marathon runner may have to try shorter distances such as half-marathons or 10-kilometre races, and training may have to be adjusted to include less running mileage and more protective conditioning work. The weight-trainer may have to leave out exercises involving deep knee bending movements, and change from lifting heavy weights to doing more or faster repetitions with lighter weights. If it is not possible to continue sport without making the osteoarthritic pain worse, it may be better for the sports participant to take up new types of exercise, such as swimming or cycling, to avoid the frustration and physical disadvantage of giving up sport altogether, and to minimise the risk of sudden weight increase.

Osteoarthritic pain can be treated in the first instance by physiotherapy techniques, which aim to reduce the pain and to improve the knee joint mechanics. Alternative treatments, such as naturopathy, acupuncture, reflexology or healing can all contribute some benefit in alleviating long-standing pain. The doctor may offer various forms of anti-inflammatory treatment. In the long term, if the condition becomes intolerable, the orthopaedic surgeon may be able to help with corrective surgery, aiming either to improve the joint mechanics, or to eliminate the pain completely by replacing the worn out joint with a new artificial one. The knee replacement operation, although not yet as commonplace as the hip replacement, is being used more often now that modern research is developing satisfactory artificial joints which can substitute for the knee's complicated mechanics.

11 Injuries to Sides and Back of the Knee

MEDIAL LIGAMENT INJURIES

Traumatic injuries can damage the medial ligament on the inner side of the knee, disrupting the central part of the ligament, or its attachment point onto the bones at either end of the ligament. A force which bends the knee sideways and separates the bones on the inner side of the joint, can overstretch or tear the medial ligament. This is called a valgus force, and it can happen in a fall with the leg stretched out sideways when a weight, such as an opponent in football, falls on the outer side of the knee. It can also happen to a pedestrian crossing the road, if a car bumper hits the outer side of the leg, while the foot stays on the ground. Twisting stresses which turn the foot outwards can damage the medial ligament. The foot can be on the ground, as in a fall on icy streets when the foot slips away, a skid while sprinting and turning in a field sport or court game, or when studs get stuck in heavy mud as a footballer is about to take a kick. Sometimes the leg is not bearing the body's weight when the medial ligament is injured, as in a ski-ing fall when the end of the ski gets caught and forces the knee to turn outwards.

The damage done may range from a minor strain of a few of the ligament's fibres, to a major break in the ligament's structure. Medial ligament injuries are normally classified in three categories. A first-degree injury involves some pain over the ligament, but little or no interference with the knee's movements. The second-degree injury disrupts some of the knee's function, and causes more noticeable pain. The third-degree injury is the most serious, including complete or partial rupture in the ligament, causing serious impairment of knee function.

Overuse injuries can affect the medial ligament, particularly in association with activities which repetitively bend and twist

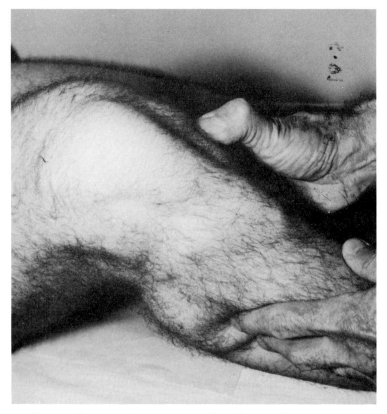

Feeling (palpating) the inner joint line for tenderness

the knee. The problem is so common among competitive swimmers with slight technique faults that it is often called 'breast-stroker's knee'. Attritional over-stretching of the medial ligament can happen through forcing the stretching movements which bend and twist the knee, such as the 'frog' stretch (Bhekasana) or the Virasana postures in Yoga. Karate players risk a similar injury when they stretch the inner thigh muscles by gradually spreading their feet apart while holding another person on their shoulders: the heavy loading means that even a slight over-stretch is likely to pull the medial ligaments. In everyday life the medial ligament can be subjected to overuse strains through long periods of sitting with the knees tucked sideways under the body, a favourite posture among children and teenagers when they watch television or listen to music.

Pain in medial ligament injuries is felt over the damaged part when the ligament is put under stress, for instance if the leg is pulled sideways to bend the knee inwards, or if the foot is twisted outwards. Walking may be painful, especially if the knee twists slightly as it goes forwards with the foot off the ground. Squatting or straightening the knee out hard may cause pain, depending on which part of the ligament is injured. Running in a straight line may still be possible in a minor injury, but twisting and turning movements are too painful. The ligament is usually tender to touch, if it is pressed along its line with the knee slightly bent. There may be swelling and bruising over the ligament in a traumatic injury, while the overuse injury usually shows no external signs of damage. Sometimes the pain of a traumatic injury only appears some hours after the accident, so that a games player, for instance, may be able to finish the match and go home before becoming aware of the damage. When the ligament is completely ruptured, the pain may not be extreme, but the knee usually feels lax or unstable, especially when the foot is off the ground.

First-aid for the traumatic injury consists of ice applications and a padded bandage which holds the knee as straight as possible. The victim should try to do knee-straightening movements or knee-cap twitching exercises immediately, if the pain is not too great. The traumatic injury may cause damage to other structures besides the medial ligament. As it is attached to the medial cartilage (meniscus), the cartilage may be torn when the ligament goes. Forced sideways movements may cause bone fracture if the ligament holds or tears only partly: this is especially common in children and teenagers, as the epiphyses (growing ends) of their shin- and thigh-bones are often weaker against applied forces than the medial ligament. A less severe force may damage the pes anserinus tendons together with the medial ligament.

The doctor, casualty officer or orthopaedic surgeon examining the knee establishes first of all how much damage has been done. If the medial ligament alone is injured, treatment for the minor injury usually consists of protecting the knee in a bandage or cast while it is acutely painful, and then regaining active function, usually under the supervision of a physiotherapist. For the second degree injury, the knee is usually protected for much longer, sometimes up to six weeks, in a plaster cast, firm bandage or brace. Alternatively, the doctor may decide to inject the ligament to reduce its pain and inflammation, and then initiate an active recovery programme, encouraging early movement through physiotherapy. For the third degree injury, the surgeon tests the medial ligament to see whether it is completely ruptured, by pulling the knee sideways to show up the abnormal gap on the inner side. Sometimes this test has to be done under anaesthetic, if the knee is too painful. The surgeon has to decide whether surgery is necessary to repair the ruptured ligament, and he then dictates the phases of recovery. In all cases the patient is asked to start doing isometric straight-leg exercises immediately (pp. 24–27). In no circumstances is knee movement, especially bending, forced.

One complication of traumatic medial ligament tears at the upper bone attachment is Pellegrini-Stieda's 'disease', which is the formation of bone particles at the point where the tendon has been torn. These bone chips can limit the knee's bending movement, hindering the recovery of knee function. They are more likely to form if the ligament has been irritated by rubbing or forced movements. Once they are present, the knee is treated very carefully, and slowly progressed towards full function. It is rare for surgeons to remove the bone chips, as they tend to re-form. Any traumatic medial ligament injury may take up to three months for full recovery; the severe injury, or a more minor one which has developed Pellegrini-Stieda's condition, can take up to a year to regain full function. If recovery is likely to be slow, a supportive brace may be used to allow safe movement in the knee, and this may even make some sports participation possible.

Overuse medial ligament injuries can be very slow to heal, if they have developed into chronic problems. Once the doctor or orthopaedic specialist has ruled out the possibility of disease, bone damage, or any other possible cause of similar pain, treatment may consist of an injection or various physiotherapy modalities, coupled with progressive exercises to build up the knee's protection through its muscles (pp. 24 and 38). All the knee's muscle groups are important in this, but special emphasis may be placed on the inner thigh muscles (adductors) in conjunction with the quadriceps (for instance, no. 11 p. 26). Twisting movements are avoided for as long as they cause pain. A brace may be used to protect the knee from sideways stresses. If the overuse injury is treated early, and protected from painful movements, recovery can be relatively quick, but the chronic, established problem can take up to a year, or more.

LATERAL LIGAMENT INJURIES

The lateral ligament, binding the outer side of the knee, is not as easily injured as the medial (inner side) ligament. Traumatically, the lateral ligament can be injured if the knee is forced outwards relative to the shin- and thigh-bones. This can happen in a sideways fall, especially if the foot gets caught as the knee gives way. Footballers and rugby players are vulnerable to this injury if they fall sideways in a tackle and another player falls onto the inner side of the injured leg, increasing the sideways pressure on it.

If the force of the injury is severe enough, other structures besides the lateral ligament may be injured, and there is a lot of pain and swelling over the knee. The examining doctor will check for signs of cartilage or cruciate ligament damage. When the lateral ligament is injured on its own, in a moderately severe injury, the doctor may recommend ice applications, support bandaging and rest from any stressful activities, and he is likely to refer the patient for physiotherapy treatment to help restore good muscle function in the knee. One complication of the lateral ligament tear that the doctor will watch for is damage to the nerve which lies close to the ligament at the side of the knee, the lateral popliteal nerve. Damage to this nerve causes a 'dropped foot', an inability to draw the foot upwards from the ankle, so that the foot drags during walking. It may be necessary for the victim to wear a special foot support for a time, to make walking easier. Sitting with legs crossed has to be avoided, as this can cause extra pressure on the nerve and its blood supply, and aggravate the problem. If it is evident that the nerve has been badly torn in the injury, the doctor may decide to have it repaired surgically. If the nerve is partly damaged or over-stretched the physiotherapist may be able to help maintain good function in the leg until the nerve recovers.

The lateral ligament can also suffer overuse strains if the knee is thrown off balance so that its outer side is over-stretched. One common cause of this is poor foot mechanics in which the foot rolls outwards, or supinates, too much. This can happen through walking with a limp, with the weight on the outer side of the foot. Runners can experience the problem through running on camber, or through running in shoes which have worn down excessively on the outer sides of the soles. The problem is not usually severe, and therefore it may not need treatment, other than correction of any mechanical imbalance affecting the feet, perhaps ice applications to ease any soreness, and general knee exercises to maintain good strength and mobility in the joint (pp. 24 and 35).

ILIOTIBIAL TRACT INJURIES

The iliotibial tract, the strong band which extends down the outer side of the thigh to the side of the knee, can be injured traumatically, when the bent knee is subjected to a sudden violent movement which twists it to turn the foot and shin inwards relative to the thigh-bone. This can happen in a fall, especially if the foot gets caught during a turning movement. Players in field sports may suffer the injury on changing direction suddenly, especially during tackles, or when the playing surface is slippery or muddy.

If the tract is injured on its own, pain is felt at the side of the knee. As it is stressed, the tract can pull away, or avulse, the point of bone to which it is attached at the side of the shin-bone. There is usually some swelling, even in a minor injury. In a more serious injury, there may be damage to other structures besides the iliotibial tract, such as the lateral ligament, or internal structures like the cruciate ligaments or the cartilages (menisci), so the swelling and pain are severe, and the victim is treated as an emergency. For the minor injury, the doctor should be consulted as soon as possible. He may refer the patient to an orthopaedic specialist. Once the iliotibial tract injury is identified, the doctor or surgeon may decide to treat it by injection, or, if there is persistent swelling, he may draw off, or aspirate, the fluid, and then protect the knee in a plaster cast for about four weeks. Static exercises (pp. 24–27) are performed to maintain the leg muscles while the cast is on, and then the knee is re-strengthened and mobilised until it is fully recovered.

Overuse injury to the iliotibial tract at the side of the knee is a problem usually associated with repetitive activities or sports, such as trekking, marathon running, or cross-country ski-ing. Pain develops at the side of the knee, caused by repetitive friction. This condition is called the iliotibial tract friction syndrome. The problem is usually triggered by some change in normal activities, such as an unusually long walk, run or ski; walking or running on hills and slopes, or a particular camber;

walking or running in badly balanced shoes; walking or running with a limp from another leg or back injury; or walking or running too soon after a hip or ankle injury.

The injury causes a localised painful spot at the side of the knee, which tends to hurt only after a certain time during the pain-causing activity, for instance after about twenty minutes' running. Once the pain starts, it continues as long as the activity is continued, but it subsides almost immediately when the activity stops, and it is not normally noticeable at other times. Sometimes there is a pocket of swelling at the side of the knee, and a painful spot on pressure. The pain is caused by damage under the iliotibial tract: there may be irritation on the inner side of the tract itself; or the bursa, the fluid-filled sac which lies under the tract, may become an inflamed cyst.

The doctor who examines the knee needs an accurate account of how the pain began and developed. He can usually locate the tender point in this friction syndrome, by bending the knee to about thirty degrees and pressing on the side of the iliotibial tract with his thumb. He may be able to feel a snapping sensation if he bends and straightens the knee passively, keeping his thumb over the sore spot. If there is any doubt about the diagnosis, further checks may be ordered, such as X-rays. Once the diagnosis is established, the doctor may treat the problem with anti-inflammatory drugs, an injection into the painful spot, or he may refer the patient for physiotherapy treatment. If the problem has developed to a severe stage, orthopaedic surgery is the last resort for clearing the inflamed area.

In most cases, rest from the activity which caused the problem is recommended, while a treatment programme is carried out. However, if necessary, it may be possible to continue some training, with modifications aimed at preventing the pain from recurring or, at least, getting worse. For instance, a runner may be able to train over shorter distances, perhaps running faster than normal, doing shuttle runs to vary the stresses on the knee, running clockwise on the track, or running on different surfaces. The runner may also be able to run in shallow water in the swimming pool. Using different shoes may help, or, if a foot mechanics defect has contributed to the problem, orthotics from a podiatrist may allow painless walking and running. Meanwhile, the knee muscles must be maintained, with special emphasis on strengthening the muscles over the front and outer side of the knee through static exercises (pp. 24–27) and perhaps weight-resisted exercises (p. 35). The outer side of the knee should also be stretched frequently each day, and especially before and after any exercise session (p. 35, nos 9 and 10). Normal sports training should be resumed gradually, once the problem is cured. Recurrence should be avoided through awareness of the injury's cause.

TIBIOFIBULAR JOINT INJURIES

The superior (upper) tibiofibular joint, just below the outer side of the knee, can be injured traumatically. A direct blow to the top of the fibula can dislocate the joint forwards or backwards, especially if the knee is bent. This can be a kick in football or a blow from a hockey stick. A sudden contraction of the biceps tendon can pull the head of the fibula backwards, for instance if a hamstring curl exercise is too heavy in weight-training, or if a person trips coming down stairs and pulls up sharply to prevent a fall. A fall while walking can disrupt the joint, if the foot is caught turned in pointing downwards, and the knee is bent. Landing awkwardly from a great height can harm the joint, as in parachuting or a fall from a roof.

Testing the stability of the superior tibiofibular joint

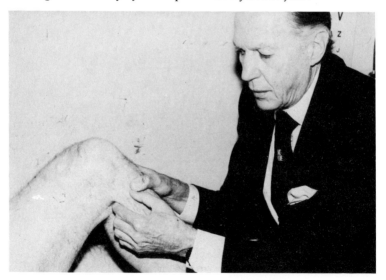

Overuse injuries are less common, but they can occur if the tibiofibular joint has been damaged previously and become lax, or if the joint is congenitally unstable, having grown with loose ligaments. The problem is relatively more common in young active people than in the elderly. The joint may dislocate or sublux apparently without warning when the leg is being used at a particular angle, for instance when the victim is running on bends on a track, getting up from squatting, or sitting with one leg crossed over the other. If the joints are congenitally loose, both may tend to give way, separately or together. The injury tends to be recurrent, usually becoming gradually worse each time.

The damaged tibiofibular joint causes pain and sometimes swelling over the outer side of the knee. If the dislocation is bad enough, there may be a visible deformity, with the top of the fibula jutting out. If the joint subluxes, the victim may feel that the fibula 'pops' momentarily. The joint may be tender to touch. Occasionally the joint's disruption affects the nerve that lies close to the top of the fibula, called the common peroneal nerve, and this causes tingling or numbness in the nerve's pathway down the lower leg. Usually the normal knee movements of bending and straightening cause no additional pain, although squatting or twisting the knee may.

Bad injuries to the tibiofibular joint often cause more extensive damage to the knee joint or the knee bones, so the examining doctor has to sort out priorities and deal with the most serious aspects, such as bone fractures, cartilage tears or cruciate ligament damage, first. Sometimes, the tibiofibular joint injury is overlooked in the first instance, and this can be one reason why it develops into a recurrent problem later. If the tibiofibular joint is injured on its own, treatment depends on the severity of the damage. For a minor sprain, the doctor may choose to inject the ligaments, to reduce their inflammation and pain. Physiotherapy treatment may help to restore full movement and muscle stability to the joint. If the joint is dislocated, it may be manipulated back into place, and then protected in a plaster cast. If it is badly disrupted, surgery may be necessary to restore its stability.

124. Injuries to Sides and Back of the Knee

MUSCLE AND TENDON INJURIES ON THE BACK OF THE KNEE

Traumatic strains and tears can occur in the muscles and tendons at the back of the knee. If the knee is forced backwards, the back of the knee may be over-stretched: this can happen in a fall with the leg outstretched, especially if extra pressure is applied over the front of the knee, such as an opponent falling onto the leg in a football tackle. Over-kicking in football or karate can pull the back of the knee. Over-contraction can also cause sudden injury to the muscles and tendons, for instance during a fall backwards where the foot is blocked, or a hamstring curl exercise in weight-training using too much load.

Overuse injuries can affect the muscles and tendons at the back of the knee. Gradually increasing pain can be associated with awkward movements with the knee held bent, for instance the twisting while crouching or kneeling that a carpet-layer, electrician or plumber might have to do while working at floor level. Sports such as fencing, squash and rowing which involve repeated knee bending movements can cause overuse strains, often through faulty foot movements which cause slight variations in the twisting stresses on the knee. The muscles and tendons can also tighten or stiffen, without any direct injury. Whenever the knee is injured, whether inside the joint or over the front of it, there is an immediate inhibition of the quadriceps muscles which straighten the knee, especially vastus medialis which locks it out. This is accompanied by a reflex tightening or spasm at the back of the knee, which is a protective mechanism to hold the knee in a slightly bent position in order to minimise its pain. A similar mechanism occurs when the knee suffers from degenerative, or wear-and-tear, arthritis. Sometimes the first sign of the condition is a gradual stiffening of the knee as the tendons at the back pull the knee into the slightly bent position. The tightness can also be brought on through postural habits, such as sitting for long periods with the knees bent, or wearing high-heeled shoes most of the time. Many sports can cause similar knee stiffness, such as sprinting and squash. In childhood and the early teenage years, the combination of a sport which works the knee in the bent position and bone growth without a parallel lengthening out of the muscles can lead to shortening of all the muscles at the back of the leg, and a severe limitation of knee extension.

Injuries to the back of the knee can affect the hamstring tendons, the gastrocnemius tendons or the popliteus muscle and its tendon. In a traumatic injury, damage may range from a minor strain of some fibres to a total tear, or rupture, of the injured structure. Overuse injuries may involve strains or minor tears; popliteal bursitis, or inflamed cysts under the tendons; or, in the case of popliteus, tenosynovitis, or inflammation in the fluid-filled lining surrounding the popliteus tendon. Pain is felt when the injured area is put on the stretch, as when the knee is straightened fully. Working the injured muscles or tendons causes pain. If the hamstring tendons are injured, they may cause pain walking down stairs, or walking and turning to one side. The gastrocnemius tendons cause pain particularly during running, especially on a track or up stairs. The popliteus muscle causes pain during squatting, and when the knee is bent and twisted inwards against a resistance, for instance in using the foot to scratch the front of the uninjured leg. In a traumatic injury, there may be bruising and swelling around the injury, and the area may be very tender to touch at first. A bursitis may cause a visible egg-like swelling at the back of the knee, although it is not necessarily painful. Sometimes, a bursitis keeps occurring under the semimembranosus or gastrocnemius tendons on the inner side of the back of the knee: this can become a chronic, repetitive condition, and it has a special name, 'Baker's cyst'.

First-aid for the traumatic injury consists of ice applications to limit the pain, swelling and bruising, and protection from any painful activities. A bandage may be used for comfort, and in a severe injury the victim may need to be carried off, although more often walking is still possible. The examining doctor usually checks whether any internal joint structures, such as the cartilages (menisci) or cruciate ligaments have been injured as well as the muscles or tendons. Testing the muscles and tendons by making them contract to bend and twist the knee against the resistance of the doctor's hand shows up their pain. Localised tender spots may be felt when the doctor presses over the back of the knee with the patient lying prone. The popliteus tendon may be tender just over the outer side of the knee, with the patient sitting with his knee bent and relaxed out sideways, and his foot resting over the uninjured leg. If the damage is localised to the muscles or tendons, physiotherapy treatment is usually recommended, partly to reduce the pain and swelling, and mainly to help regain full flexibility and power in the injured structures.

In the overuse injury, the doctor needs a clear picture of how the pain started. Investigations such as X-rays, arthrograms or blood tests may be needed to help establish the diagnosis. If the injury is a tendon or muscle strain with one particularly painful spot, the doctor may inject it. Physiotherapy treatment aims to help regain full function. It is particularly important to stretch the back of the knee by using exercises such as nos 1, 2, 5 and 6 on pp. 33–34. If there is a recurrent cyst at the back of the knee, the doctor may refer the patient to an orthopaedic surgeon, with a view to having it removed.

Index